HEALTHY FOODS DURING PREGNANCY:

Healthy Whole Diets for Pregnant and Breastfeeding Women

Susan J. Holt

Table of Contents

CHAPTER 1

FIRST TRIMESTER OF PREGNANCY

A Few Words on Due Dates and Trimesters

After you announce your pregnancy, the first question you'll undoubtedly be asked is "When are you due?" At your first prenatal appointment, your health care physician will help you calculate an estimated delivery date (EDD). Your EDD is 40 weeks from the first day of your last menstrual period (LMP) (LMP).

It's crucial to remember that your due date is merely an estimate - most infants are born between 38 and 42 weeks from the first day of their mom's LMP and only a tiny number of women deliver on their due date.

Another popular phrase you'll hear during your pregnancy is trimester. Pregnancy is split into trimesters:

the first trimester is from week 1 to the end of week 12, the second trimester is from week 13 to the end of week 26, and the third trimester is from week 27 to the conclusion of the pregnancy

What to Eat in the First Trimester

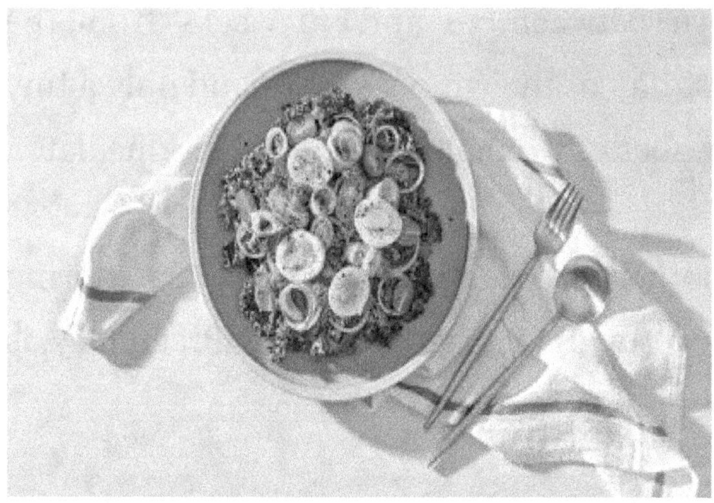

Early pregnancy sickness, food aversions, and weariness all make 'eating for two' hardship in the first trimester of pregnancy.

Between the morning sickness and heartburn, eating healthy may have gone off your to-do list during the first trimester of pregnancy.

Your body is experiencing a rise in hormones right now, which may contribute to nausea. The hormone progesterone in particular may produce digestive pain, including constipation and indigestion.

In early pregnancy, many moms-to-be discover that they have little desire to consume some of the healthful items they used to adore, such as fresh vegetables or lean meats. (Don't panic - for many pregnant women, hunger comes back in the second trimester.)

For now, don't stress it too much if you're not in the mood to fill up a full plate for every meal. Instead, concentrate on these good-for-you meals in the first trimester to cover your nutritional bases.

How many more calories do you need during the first trimester?

During the first trimester, your baby's energy demands — like your baby! — are still fairly few. You should try to consume around 2,000 calories a day in the first trimester, but your practitioner may prescribe more depending on your activity level. This amount is quite on pace with usual adult dietary recommendations.

Aim to consume three meals a day, plus one or two snacks. If you're having difficulties with portion sizes, focus on quality - making sure that the food you do manage to get down is both healthy and tastes good to you at that time. (We understand it: Sometimes what you're desiring or what you can stomach changes throughout pregnancy hour by hour.)

Stick to whichever wholesome meals you find pleasant and give good first-trimester nourishment.

What nutrients do you require during the first trimester?

Aim to load up on important pregnant nutrients during the following nine months, but in the first trimester, concentrate in particular on:

- Folic acid: This is the most crucial element in terms of first-trimester nutrition — and prenatal nutrition in general. That's because folic acid (also known as vitamin B9 or folate, when it's in dietary form) plays a critical role in preventing neural tube abnormalities. To obtain the needed 600 micrograms per day, take a prenatal vitamin every day and consume oranges, strawberries, green leafy vegetables, fortified breakfast cereals, kidney beans, almonds, cauliflower, and beets.

- Protein: It's crucial for muscle development for both you and the baby, and promotes uterine tissue growth. Aim for roughly 75 grams each day. Good sources include eggs, Greek yogurt, and poultry.

- Calcium: It's vital for your baby's growing teeth and bones. Since your developing baby will consume calcium from your reserves, too little calcium in your diet might result in brittle bones (osteoporosis) later on. You can normally acquire the necessary 1,000 milligrams per day from a well-balanced diet containing milk, cheese, yogurt, and dark leafy greens, but if you're afraid you could be falling short, ask your OB/GYN whether you should take a supplement.

- Iron: Iron is especially vital when your blood supply ramps up to meet the needs of your developing kid. The target of 27 milligrams per day might be a struggle to attain via diet alone, so make sure you're taking a strong dose of iron in your prenatal vitamin to lower the risk for pregnant anemia.

Work excellent sources like steak, poultry, eggs, tofu, and spinach into your diet plan too.

- Vitamin C: C-rich foods like oranges, broccoli, and strawberries stimulate bone and tissue growth in your developing baby and enhance the absorption of iron. You should aim for 85 milligrams each day.

- Potassium: It partners up with salt to assist your body to maintain adequate fluid balance and also controls blood pressure. Aim to receive 2,900 milligrams each day with your prenatal vitamin and foods like bananas, apricots, and avocados.

- DHA: A vital omega-3 fatty acid, DHA is found in low-mercury seafood including anchovies, herring, and sardines. You may be too nauseated for seafood these days, so ask your doctor about taking a DHA supplement.

Best meals during the first trimester

Nutrition specialists suggest the following foods in particular as they're great sources of the vitamins, minerals, and macronutrients your body (and your baby's growing body) needs to flourish.

- Lean meat: A strong source of iron and protein, thoroughly-cooked lean meats like sirloin or chuck steak, pork tenderloin, turkey and chicken contain all of the amino acids that function as the building blocks for cells.

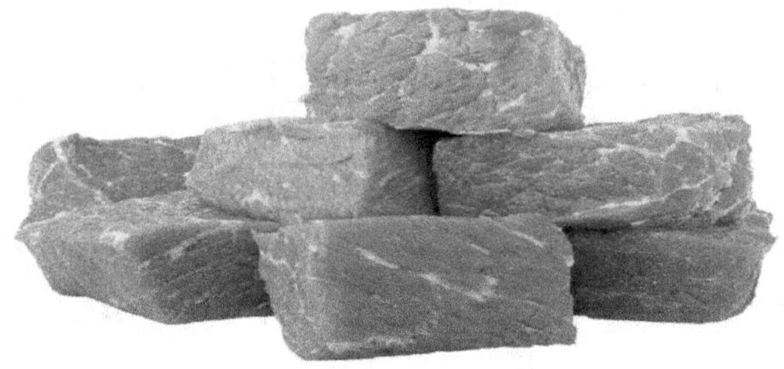

- Yogurt: The calcium and protein in each cup aid bone formation. Opt for a variety with a short ingredient list and little added sugars.

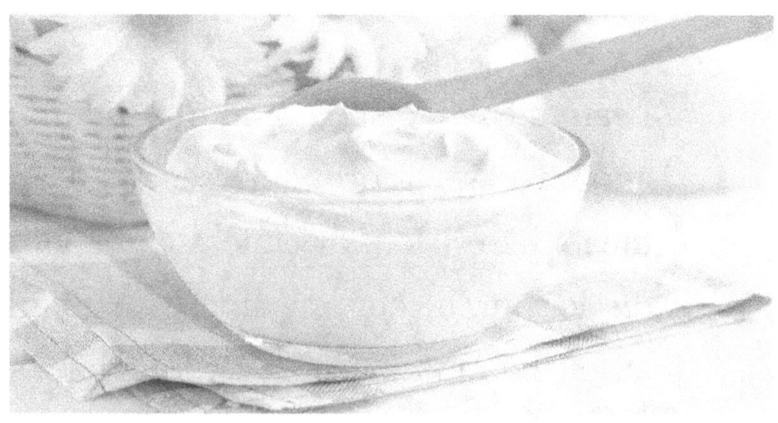

- Edamame: These soybean pods are filled with vegetarian protein, plus calcium, iron, and folate.

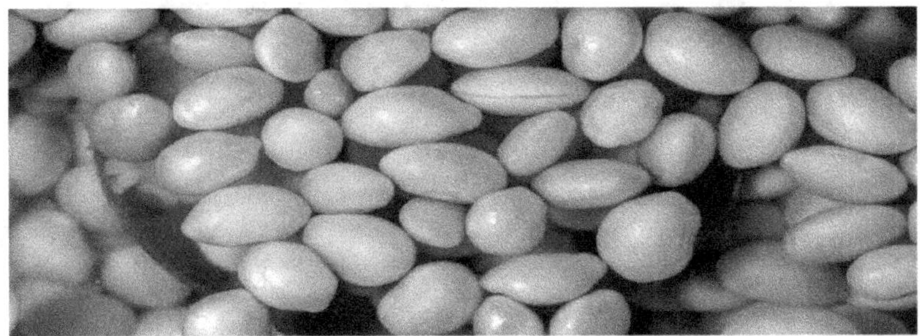

- Kale: This dark leafy green delivers a combination plate of nutrients, including fiber, calcium, folate, iron, vitamin A, vitamin C, vitamin E, and vitamin K.

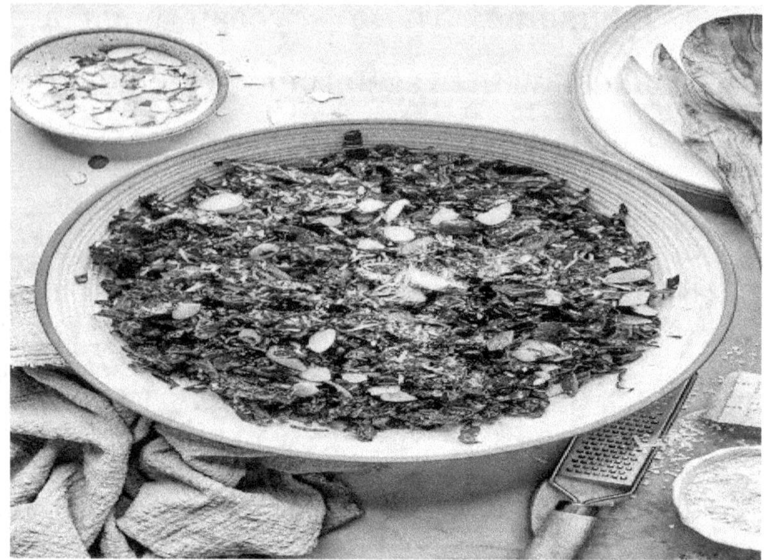

- Bananas: Bland enough to be edible for unsettled stomachs, bananas are among the finest dietary sources of potassium.

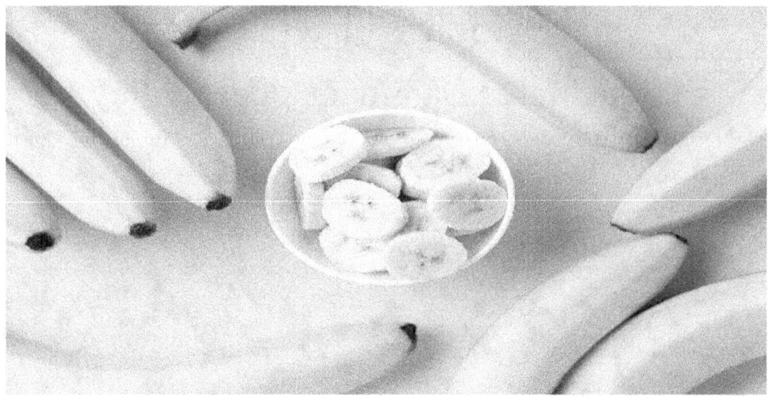

- Beans and lentils: Iron, folate, protein, and fiber are all hidden within these small-but-mighty powerhouses.

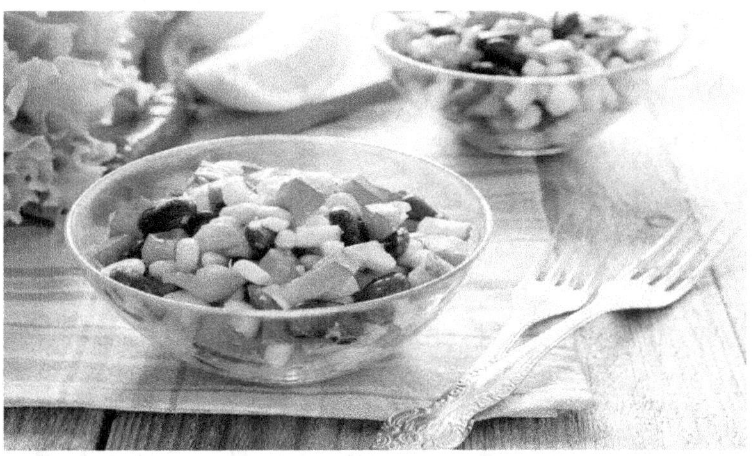

- Ginger drink: Ginger items, such as ginger tea or ginger chews, may help fight nausea.

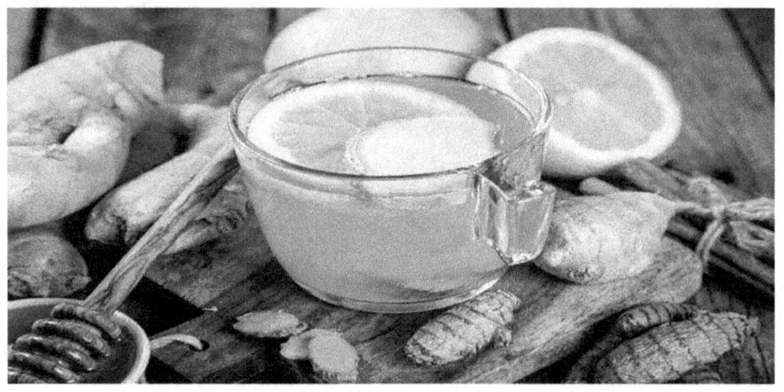

What should you consume if you're battling morning sickness and nausea?

About 75% of expecting women suffer nausea, upset stomach, or other morning sickness symptoms during the first three months of pregnancy. To attempt to relieve the case:

Fuel yourself with several little meals every few hours instead of attempting to push three large meals a day. Going too long without eating may make nausea worse, as can eating huge meals.

Avoid hot and extremely high-fat meals, since they might contribute to heartburn or stomach pain.

Stick with cold or room-temperature bland meals when you're feeling most sick, such as yogurt with fruit, string cheese with nuts, or a tiny bagel with nut butter. Hot meals are more likely to generate scents that may make nausea worse.

Try liquid or softly-textured foods. You may have an easier time digesting a homemade smoothie, oatmeal, or noodles when your stomach feels uncomfortable.

Keep dry, easy-to-eat snacks on hand, such on your nightstand and in your handbag or work bag. Graham crackers, pretzels, and low-sugar dry cereal are good grab-and-go alternatives.

First-trimester healthy eating suggestions

Ultimately, although it's vital to eat healthy throughout the first trimester, try not to worry too much about what you're putting on your plate, as this may add extra stress to a period that is likely already packed with lots of anxiety.

Although diversity is vital, you'll likely have an easier time filling your plate with a larger choice of meals if your nausea and morning sickness diminishes in the second trimester. So for now, take it easy on yourself — and your stomach. Don't forget to:

- Stay hydrated: Fill up a glass with water and leave it on your nightstand before bed, then wake up and drink it before beginning your day. If simple water doesn't seem pleasant, add a piece of lemon, cucumber, or fresh berries.
- Snack well: A frequent symptom early in pregnancy is the sudden onset of

hunger with a concomitant sense of nausea and even fullness. Keep your blood sugar consistent throughout the day by eating nutritious snacks, such as a small handful of nuts, a few whole-grain crackers with cheese, a piece of fresh fruit, or a slice of whole-grain toast with nut butter.

- Pop that prenatal: No one eats properly every single day, which is one reason why taking your prenatal vitamin is so crucial. Set an alarm on your phone as a reminder to take your vitamin each day.

When in doubt, contact your OB/GYN. He or she may counsel you on the foods and beverages to absolutely avoid during the first trimester, such as alcohol, unpasteurized dairy, and undercooked meats.

CHAPTER 2

SECOND TRIMESTER OF PREGNANCY

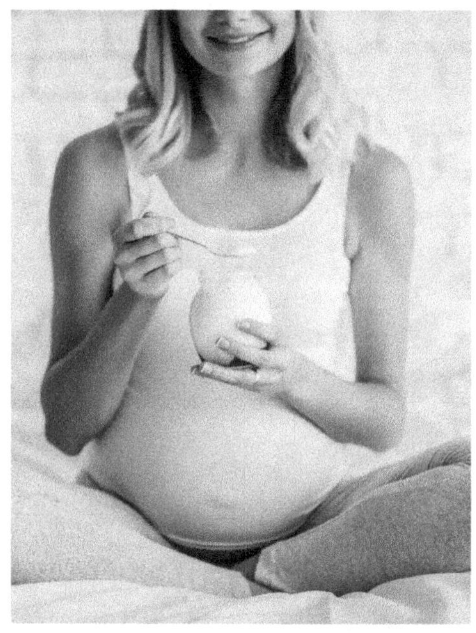

Let's discuss the second trimester! If you are approaching the second trimester, this frequently implies there is hope for the ick symptoms to begin to lessen. Perhaps, nausea/vomiting - "morning sickness", intense exhaustion, headaches, etc. will begin to lessen, and hopefully, you'll begin feeling like your old self again (with a small growing bump!).

The second trimester is characterized as weeks 13-27. While a lot occurs every week of pregnancy, this trimester is especially exciting, and you may see some of the largest physical changes occurring during this time. You will likely progress from a small little bulge to what seems like an ever-growing lovely baby bump!

What changes can I anticipate in my second trimester?

During this trimester, your tummy will be swelling and continue to develop each week as that baby becomes larger. Also, when your body is altering and developing to create space for the baby, you may begin feeling or recognizing stretch marks. While you can't avoid them, you can assist your body in preparing but lather it with moisture to help your skin prepare for development. Also, you may realize that you are a bit more hungry more frequently since your appetite is rising.

As you are seeing all of these changes and more, your baby is experiencing huge changes too. During the second trimester, your baby's organs all become entirely grown. And, during the middle to the end of the second trimester, your baby will start to wriggle and move! Exactly when you start to feel those lovely kicks is different for many women, but by the end of the second trimester, you'll be feeling your little one dance in your belly!

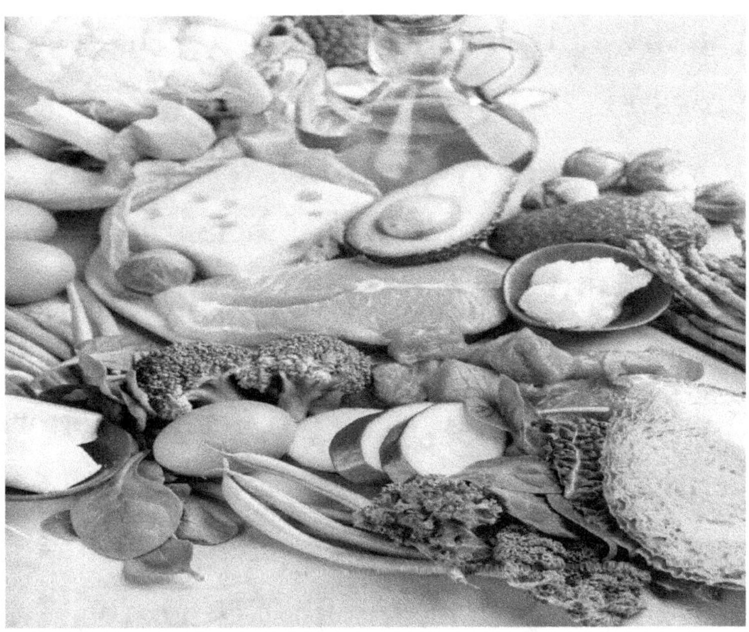

What should I be eating in my second trimester?

Moving from one trimester to another, dietary demands don't vary drastically. However, for many, getting into your second trimester also means being able to eat regularly again. Hopefully, you can eat a bit more variety when nausea decreases and you possibly have a little more energy to prepare.

If you've been able to eat balanced meals with a little amount of protein, fat, and carbohydrates with all of your meals- keep it up! If not, when you start feeling better, gently aim to eat meals with all 3 macros—focusing on quality protein, nutrient-dense fats, and fiber-rich carbs.

There are also several particular nutrients you should consider concentrating on — calcium, magnesium, vitamin D, and omega-3 fatty acids.

- Calcium: Calcium helps construct the baby's bones and teeth as well as assists in the development of the baby's musculoskeletal, neurological and circulatory systems. Fun fact: calcium absorption in your intestines increases during pregnancy, making it more accessible to you for absorption. With this, make sure you are drinking the complimentary nutrients (vitamin D, Vit K2, Mag) as well to aid with absorption. If you eat dairy products, it will be easy to make sure you're reaching your requirements. Non-dairy consumers can accomplish it, but may simply need to be more conscious about the other foods they eat. Great sources of calcium include:

- All things dairy - yogurt, cheese, and milk. Best if it is full-fat, grass-fed
- Broccoli
- Leafy Greens, including kale, collards, spinach
- Fatty seafood like sardines and salmon
- Nuts and seeds, notably almonds and chia seeds

- Magnesium: Magnesium works in combination with calcium to enhance absorption and helps establish strong bones and a neurological system for the baby. Magnesium shortage is quite common for the general population, and typically more prevalent during pregnancy. For you mommas, magnesium may help prevent or alleviate muscle cramps and aids induce relaxation. Below are a few wonderful sources of calcium:

- Green leafy vegetables
- Almonds and cashews
- Avocado
- Chia seeds
- Dark chocolate/unsweetened cocoa powder
- Epsom salt baths - you can absorb magnesium via the skin with Epsom salt baths (Epsom salt is magnesium sulfate)

(Epsom salt is magnesium sulfate)

- Vitamin D: Vitamin D also aids in bone and skeletal growth for kids in pregnancy. It also is vital for your health as a mom- low vitamin D levels have been related to an increased risk for preeclampsia, low child birth weight, and gestational diabetes. Good sources of vitamin D include:
  - Depending on where you live (exposure/closeness to the sun), a small amount of sunlight each day may be the best. It is frequently impossible to obtain all of our vitamin D from the sun owing to us being covered up with clothing, sunscreen, being

inside, cold, overcast weather, etc.

- o Salmon
- o Liver
- o Sardines
- o Fortified foods
- o Supplementation is also a fantastic alternative for vitamin D since it is hard for some of us to receive appropriate quantities or if we are deficient, practically impossible for us to get to an acceptable quantity with diet and/or sunlight alone.

- Omega-3 Fatty Acids: Omega-3 fatty acids are made up of EPA and DHA. DHA is notably crucial to the growing kid as it plays a key function in his or her brain development and protects against inflammation and damage. Good sources of Omega-3 Fatty acids include:

- o Salmon, mackerel, sardines, and trout (target of 2-3x/week)
- o Pasture-raised eggs

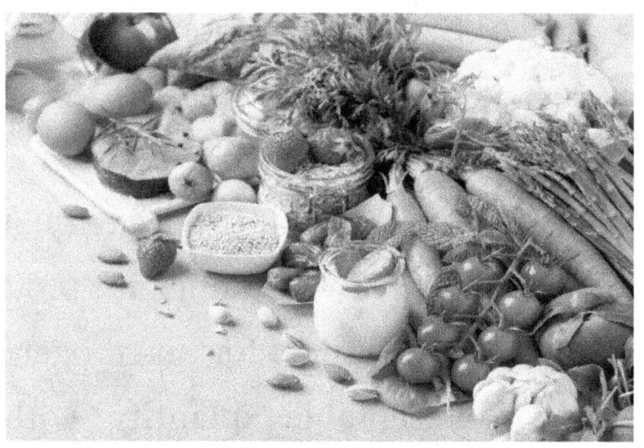

Healthy meals for your second trimester

A diversified, balanced diet, plus a vitamin D pill, should give you plenty of these nutrients. If you want some healthy suggestions to enhance your calcium and magnesium, check out these foods you may try. Make sure you and your baby are receiving all the nourishment you need with our nutritious meals particularly designed for the second trimester.

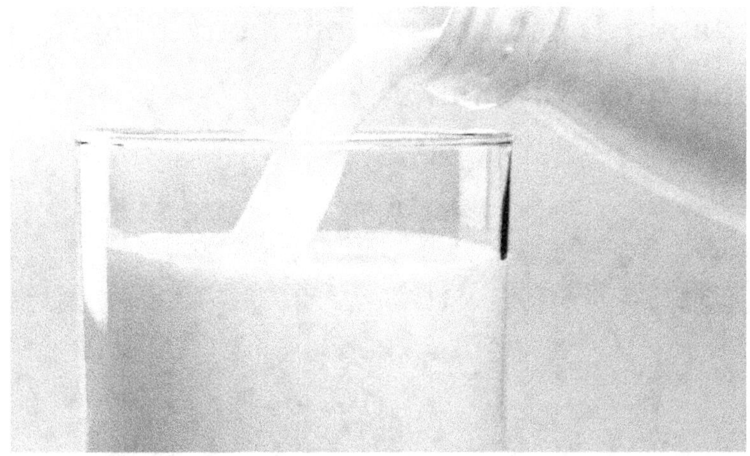

- A glass of milk: A glass of semi-skimmed milk is rich in calcium and magnesium. If you don't consume dairy products, you might try calcium-fortified soya foods, such as soya yogurts.

Keeping up your stocks of calcium during pregnancy helps your baby's bones and teeth to develop and grow strong, and a vitamin D pill assists your body to absorb and utilize calcium.

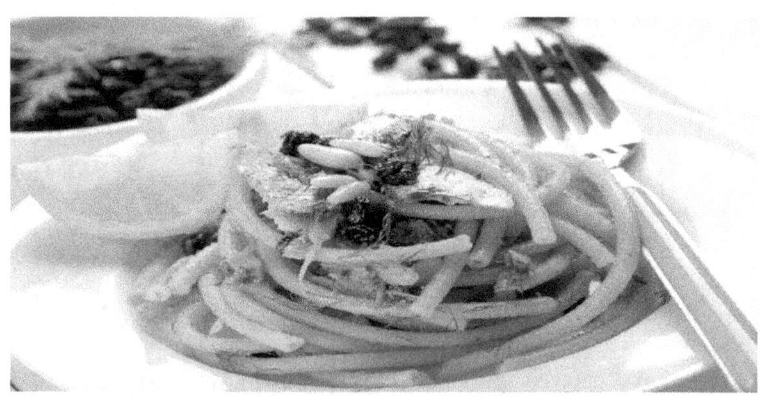

- Canned sardines: Try mashing canned sardines, including the soft, edible bones, over a piece of whole grain bread. Or sprinkle through pasta with a little parmesan and pine nuts for added magnesium and iron.

Choose sardines in oil or tomato sauce. A watercress salad is a pleasant complement that's filled with calcium and vitamin C.

Canned sardines include calcium as well as long-chain omega-3 oils and magnesium. Omega-3 oils are vital for the proper development of your baby's brain.

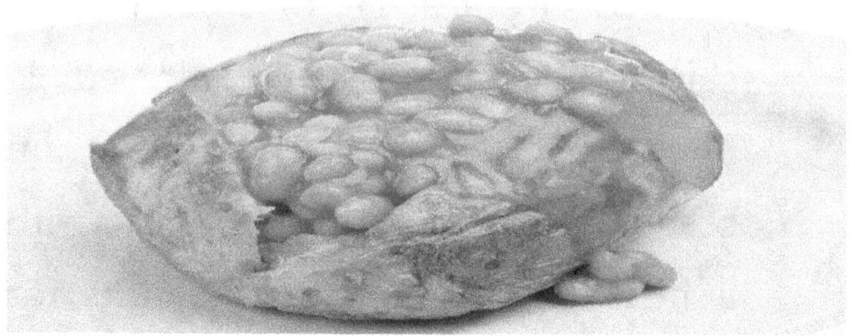

- Baked potato with beans: A jacket potato with baked beans creates magnesium, iron, and fiber-rich lunch. You may try serving this with a rocket salad to enhance vitamin C. Vitamin C enables your body to absorb iron. Magnesium is crucial for bone formation and allows your body to turn food into energy.

Iron allows you to generate red blood cells for your developing baby.

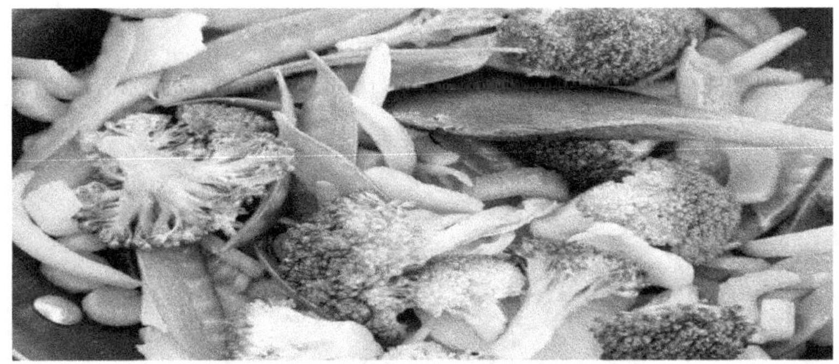

- A variety of vegetables: Use veggies that contain magnesium and calcium such as broccoli, green beans, carrots, cabbage, and okra into your meals. Stir-fry or steam to maintain the nutrients, and try not to overcook them.

Or for a snack, try crisp raw sugar snap peas, peppers, and carrots with a wonderful dip.

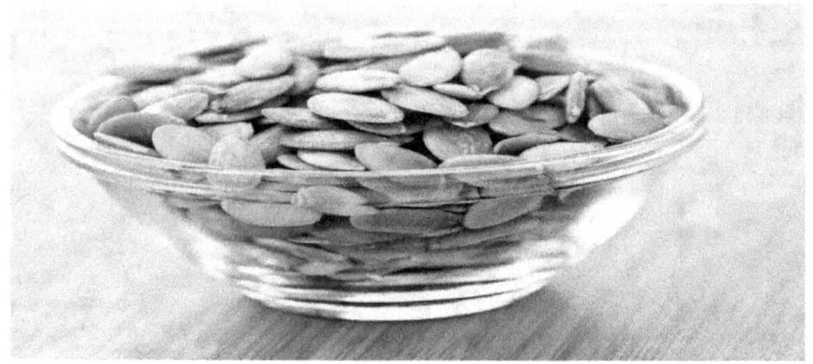

- Sunflower and pumpkin seeds: A small handful of sunflower seeds or pumpkin seeds, whether as a snack to munch or added to yogurt and salads, can provide you with magnesium, iron, and omega-3 boost.

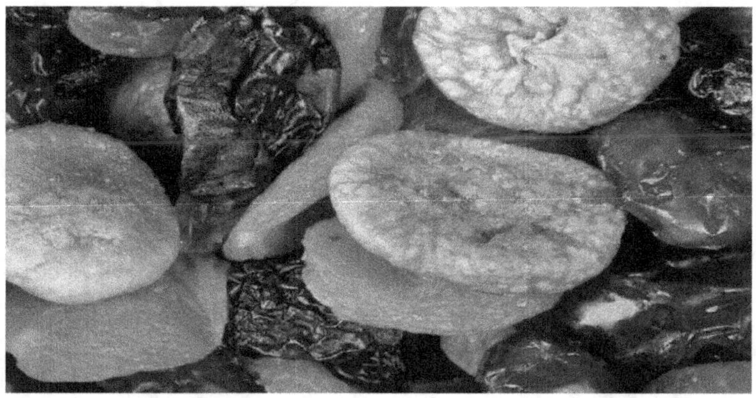

- Dried fruit: Dried fruit such as apricots, dates, and figs include calcium and iron, and are an excellent snack to keep at your desk at work or the kitchen at home for any simple grab-and-go snack. Or you might add some chopped dry fruit to low-fat yogurt.

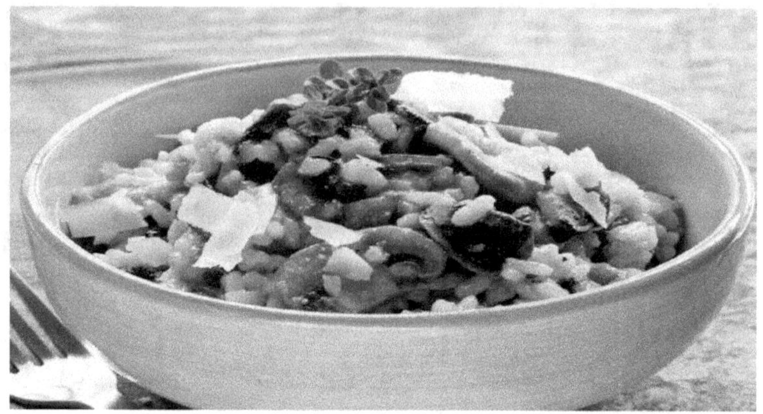

- Brown rice veggie risotto: Wholegrain or brown rice and mushrooms include magnesium, fiber, vitamin D, and calcium. Try a mushroom risotto with boiled spinach on the side, or with peas incorporated through.

The fiber will also assist to avoid pregnant constipation.

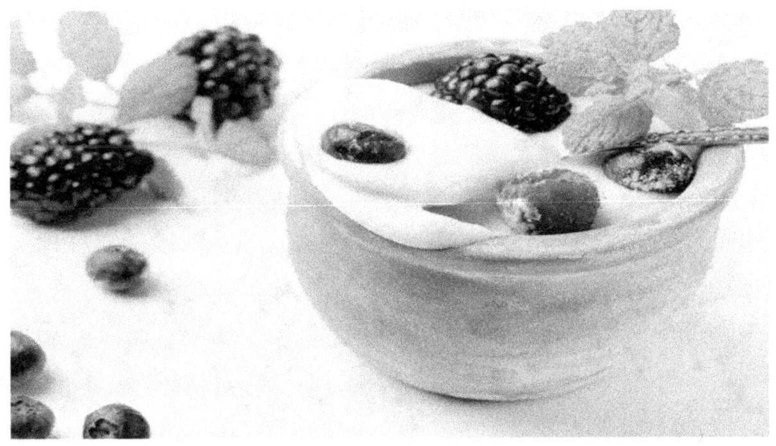

- Plain yogurt: A calcium-rich food is plain, unsweetened yogurt. Keep a pot in the fridge, or take individual pieces to work. Try low-fat Greek yogurt or fromage frais, and top with fresh fruit like blackberries, which are high in magnesium.

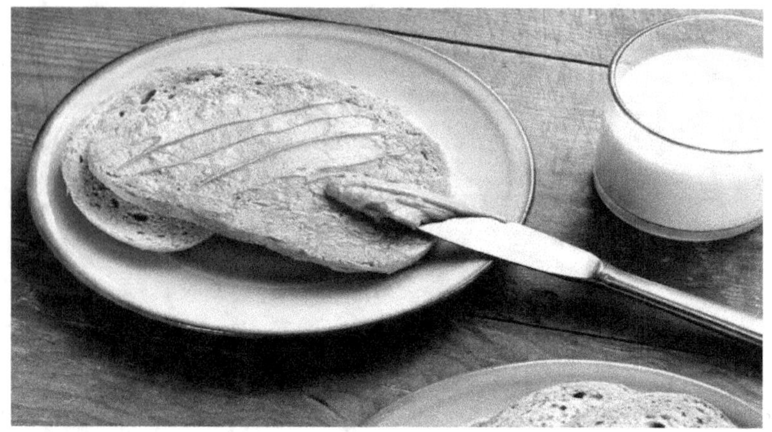

- Peanut butter on wholemeal bread: Peanut butter, or any nut butter, includes healthful fats and is a rich source of magnesium and iron, as does fortified wholegrain bread. The two combined produce a snack that will stave off any hunger sensations, and a glass of milk on the side provides calcium.

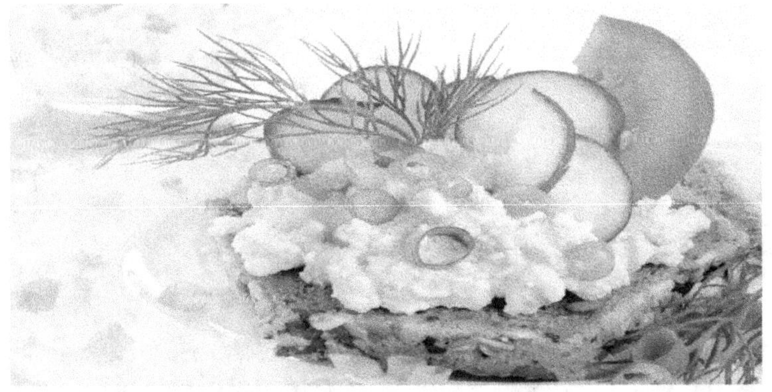

- Cheese on seeded bread: Low-fat cream cheese, or any cheese that you prefer, on seeded bread, can provide you with calcium as well as magnesium. Have with crisp salad such as radishes and cucumber.

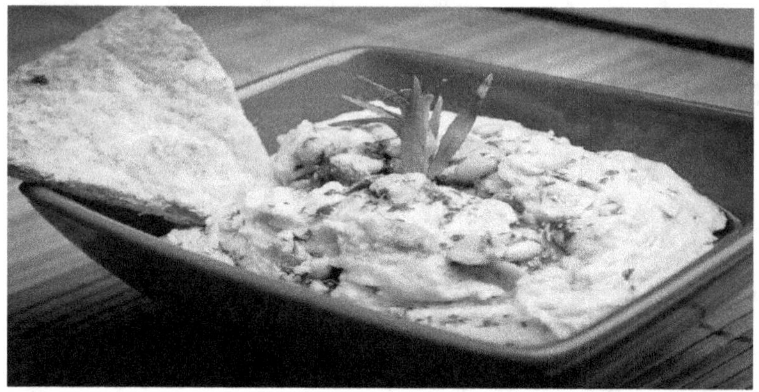

- Hummus: Have a batch of hummus in the fridge for a pleasant way to obtain calcium, magnesium, and iron. A little wholegrain pitta or granary bread and crisp raw veggies will provide magnesium.

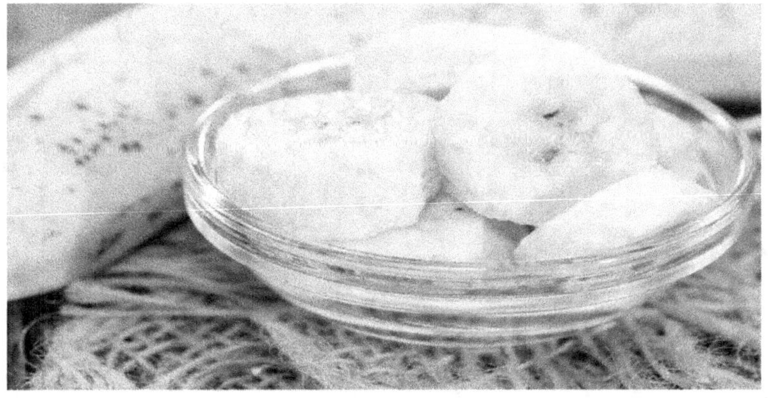

- Banana: Bananas are a wonderful source of magnesium and a quick snack for when you're busy. Try it in a smoothie, or start baking and create some banana bread.

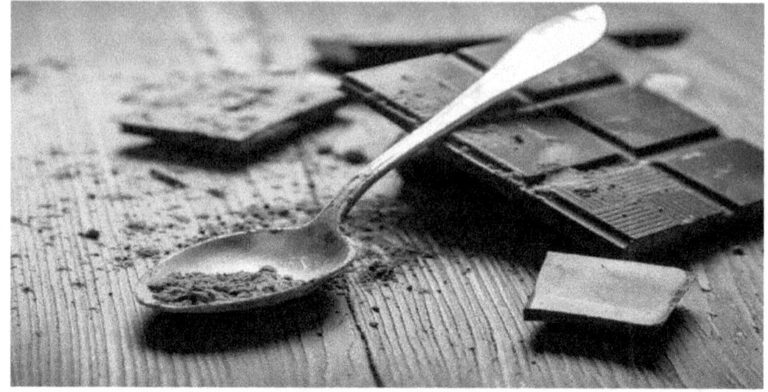

- A little dark chocolate: Believe it or not, dark chocolate includes magnesium, potassium, iron, and some calcium. Enjoy a few squares from time to time.

How much should I consume throughout my second trimester?

If you're still feeling lousy and cannot handle anything, stay in there. However, for many of us, at some time in the second trimester, we begin to feel better and may think about diversifying our diet and filling up nutrient-dense foods. Variety, color, and meals that balance all 3 macronutrients are the objective for the days and weeks ahead, concentrating on feeding that developing tiny infant.

If you are hungrier than normal, listen to it. Do not cut back, limit or worry. At no stage in pregnancy should you deny yourself sustenance? Your hunger may rise at a different rate than your friends or sisters did. Try not to compare your pregnancy to anybody else's experience or even an experience you may have had with another kid. Each pregnancy may be so diverse and taking care of our bodies and our developing infants are the focus.

If your hunger isn't revving, attempt to listen to your body. The entire concept of "eating for two" isn't exactly realistic, particularly during the second trimester. But, let us say it again - if you are hungry, eat! Choose nutrient-dense foods whether you are eating your meals or adding snacks.

What should I do about dietary intolerances during pregnancy?

Often during pregnancy, ladies can handle meals they couldn't in the past! For example, many women have reported being able to reincorporate dairy products into their diet after pregnancy.

This may be incredibly useful and a terrific way to incorporate a more diversified variety of nutrients into your diet, not to mention indulge in certain things that were previously off-limits for you! If you generally don't tolerate dairy, it may be worth trying. Just make sure that you start with a little quantity, around half the usual serving size, and work your way up from there to establish your limit.

However, it is vital to emphasize that this does not cover dietary sensitivities. If you have a real food allergy and/or a risk of an anaphylactic response, you will need to be equally as cautious as you typically are about keeping away from any allergy-inducing items. Intolerances relate to foods that induce more mild symptoms, such as stomach distress or headaches.

The second trimester is frequently described as the "best weeks of pregnancy" since for many individuals you're feeling better and your baby is developing but your increasing belly often isn't getting in the way too much or causing pain. Continue to embrace wherever you are in the pregnancy journey and try to enjoy the trip!

CHAPTER 3

THIRD TRIMESTER OF PREGNANCY

The third trimester of pregnancy spans from the 27th week to birthing. It is crucial to achieving the specified dietary needs in the third trimester to have the energy to keep up with your daily activity while supplying all necessary nutrients to your developing kid.

Previously, pregnant women were urged to eat for two, where the emphasis was focused on the amount rather than the balance of needed nutrients. The existing guidelines highlight that what you eat is more essential than how much you consume, particularly in later pregnancy.

Nutritional Requirements In Third Trimester

During the trimester, you require an extra 450 calories a day to your normal caloric and protein demands. Here are the additional nutritional details:

- DHA is necessary for the healthy development of the embryonic brain and retina throughout the third trimester. Its need rises from 100 to 200mg each day.
- You require a daily dosage of 1,000mg calcium, which is vital to create bones and teeth in your kid. Milk and other dairy products, such as cheese and

yogurt, are the finest sources of calcium.

- Vitamin D is essential for the bones to absorb calcium. You would require 15 µg per day.
- With the ongoing pregnancy, the iron needed for fetal development develops in proportion to the weight of the fetus, with most of the iron collecting during the third trimester. You would require 27mg of it every day.
- Folic acid is necessary to avert neurological abnormalities in the infant. Your consumption may go up to 800µg each day.
- You need an extra 26g a day of protein in the third trimester since it is necessary to sustain maternal tissues and fetal development.

Now that you know the number of nutrients you need, let's move into your diet plan.

Third Trimester Diet Chart

Magnesium rich foods	Dark green leafy vegetables, nuts, whole grains, avocados
Protein rich foods	Eggs, milk, yogurt, tofu, all meats
Calcium rich foods	Broccoli, watercress, cheese, seafood, dried peas, and beans
Folic acid rich foods	Lentils, beans, Brussels sprouts, oranges, eggs
Iron rich foods	Breads and pastas, beans, beets, raspberries, strawberries, red meat, dry fruits like apricots, prunes

Foods You Should Have During The Third Trimester

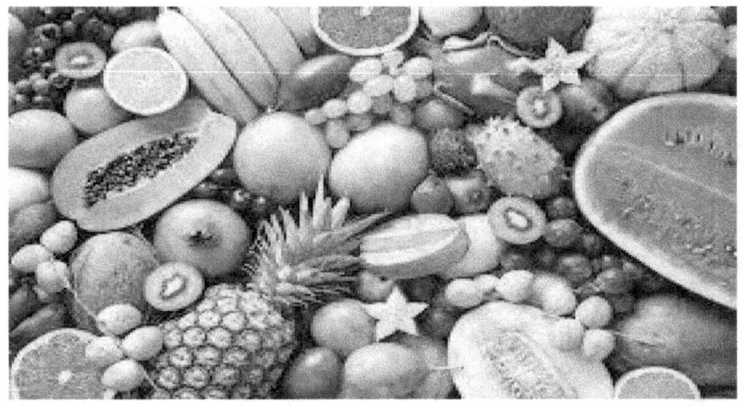

- Fruits: Fruits for nutritional needs in the third trimester.

Fresh fruits are rich in vitamin C and serve a critical role in the formation and correct functioning of the placenta. The vitamin absorbs iron from the diet and aids in keeping a robust immune system. In your third trimester, you must consume fresh fruits such as kiwis, strawberries, bananas, and melons. If you are working, then pack the fruit slices for your snacks and consume them during breaks.

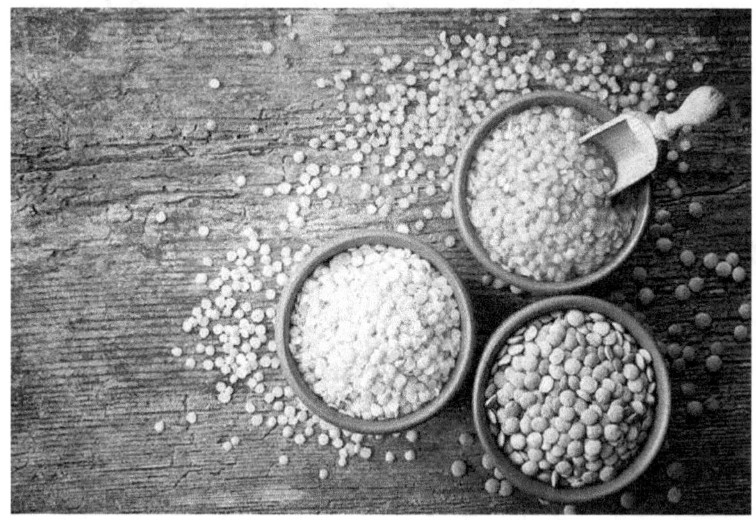

- Lentils: Lentils for nutritional needs in the third trimester.

These are high in thiamine (vitamin B1) and fiber. You may prepare soup, porridge (dal), or stew using cooked lentils and consume it in your meals.

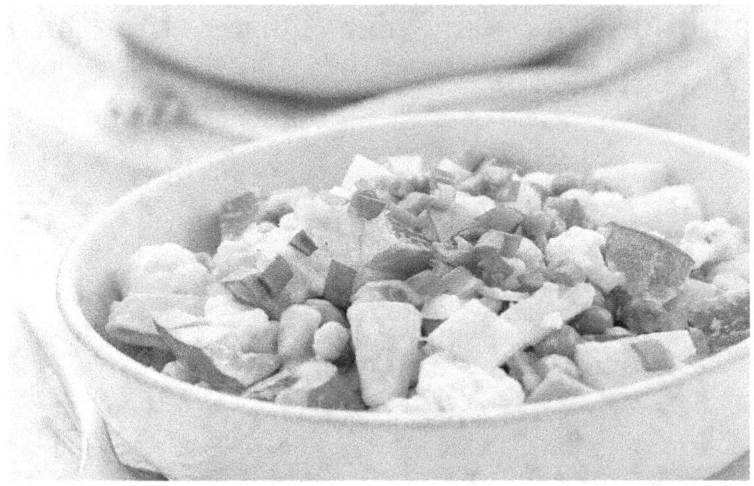

- Ham and vegetable salad: Ham and vegetable salad for nutritional needs in the third trimester

Vegetables are a good source of vitamins and ham is a thiamine booster that helps release energy from the diet. A salad of radishes, tomatoes, lettuce, and sweet corn, combined with small slices of ham, is a good addition to your diet during the third trimester.

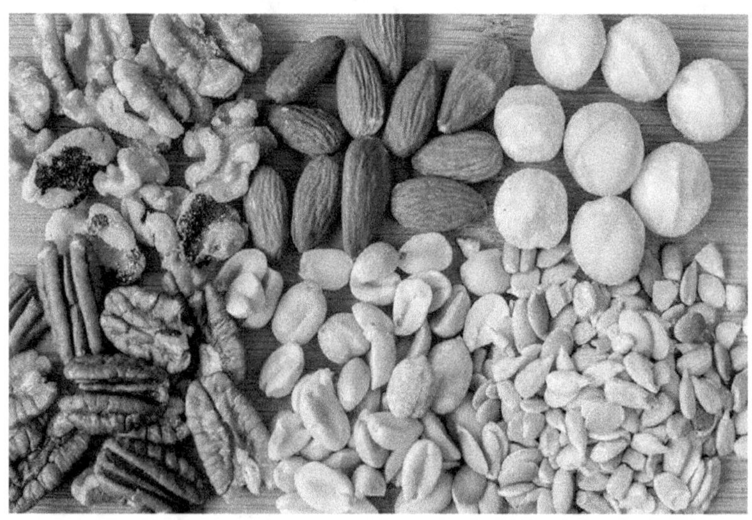

- Seeds and nuts: Seeds and nuts for nutritional needs in the third trimester

Munching on seeds and nuts will offer you with necessary levels of thiamine, important omega-3 fatty acids, and proteins. You may nibble on sunflower seeds and dry fruits such as hazelnuts, almonds, and walnuts added to your morning cereals and cereal bars.

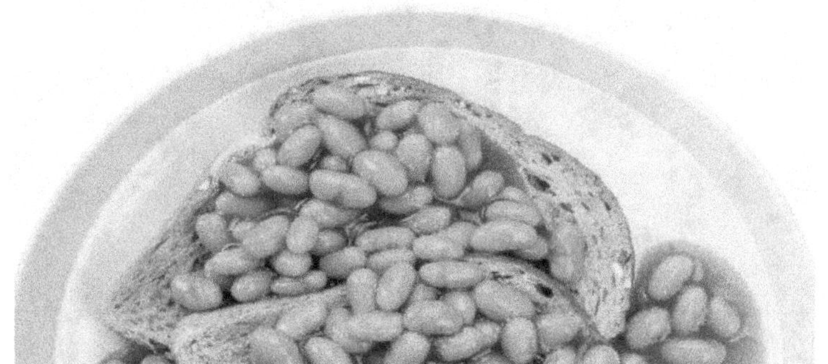

- Wholemeal toast with baked beans: Toast with baked beans for nutritional needs in the third trimester

Wholemeal toast with baked beans is high in thiamine and fiber that help maintain your energy level throughout the day and avoid constipation.

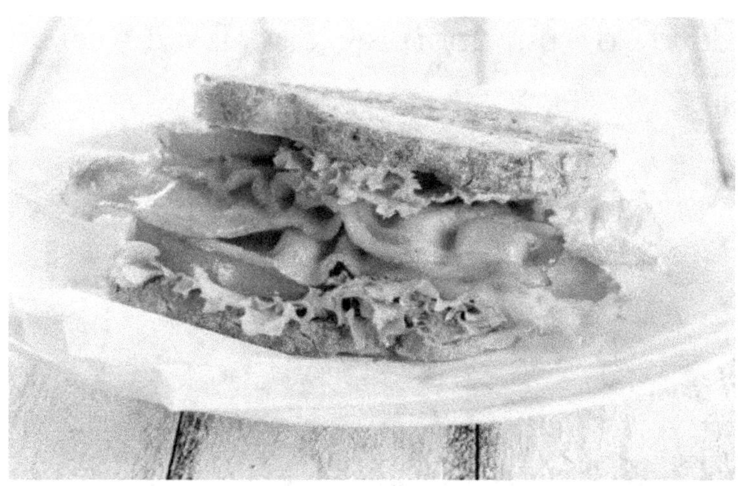

- Bacon sandwich: Bacon sandwich for nutritional needs in the third trimester

It is a power pack containing thiamine and vitamin C. Make a sandwich with thinly sliced and grilled lean bacon, sliced tomatoes, and fresh granary bread, and you will just enjoy the flavor.

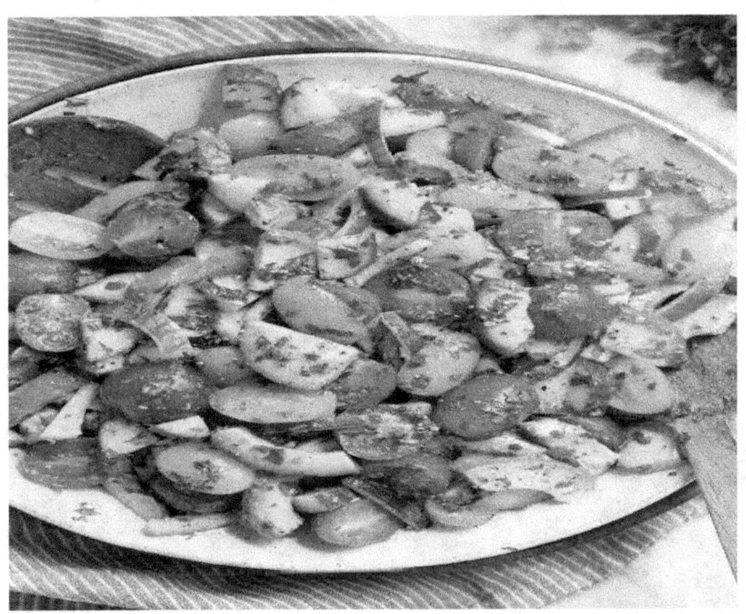

- Avocado salad: Avocado salad for nutritional needs in the third trimester

Avocado is high in vitamins C and E, as well as fiber. Mix avocado slices with walnuts, watercress, and fruits like mango or orange, and add flavorings of your choosing.

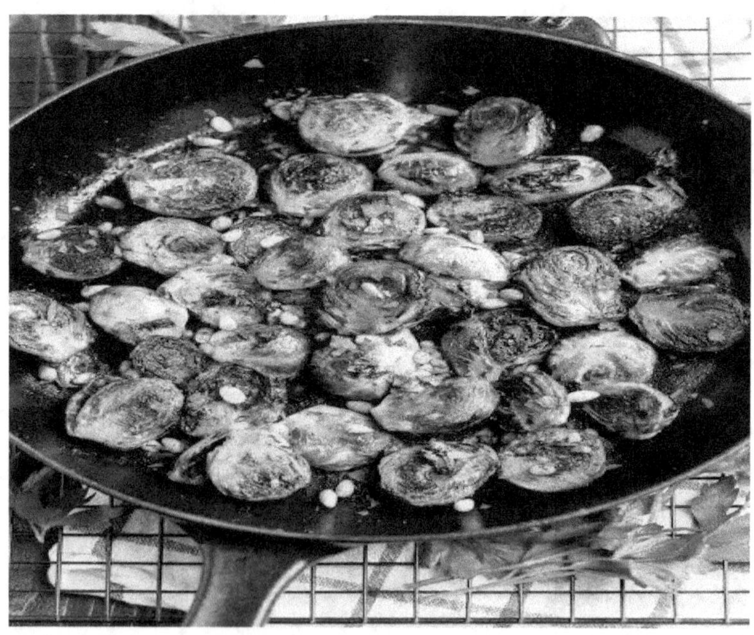

- Brussels sprouts: Brussels sprouts for nutritional needs in the third trimester

They are rich in vitamins C and K and make a fantastic side dish for your meals. It may either be steamed or microwaved till done or stir-fried with spring onions, garlic, and ginger.

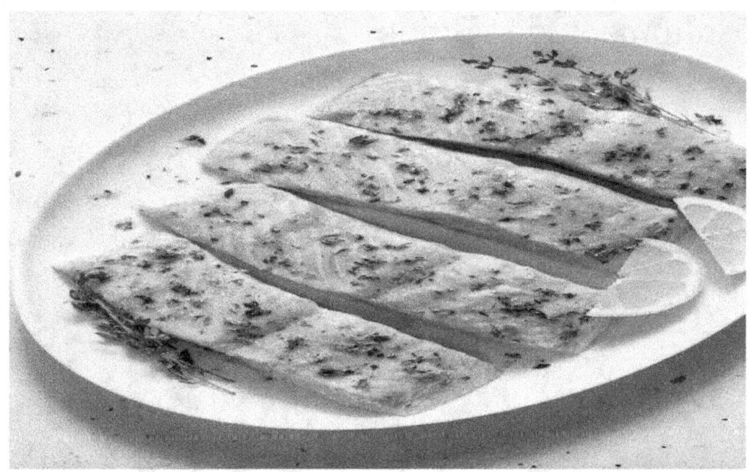

- Salmon: Salmon for nutritional needs in the third trimester

The third trimester is related to the brain development of your kid. Salmon salmon is an excellent source of omega-3 fatty acids and DHA, which is vital for the development of your baby's neurological system. However, you may take salmon in restricted amounts and only if it is well prepared. Go for homemade salmon.

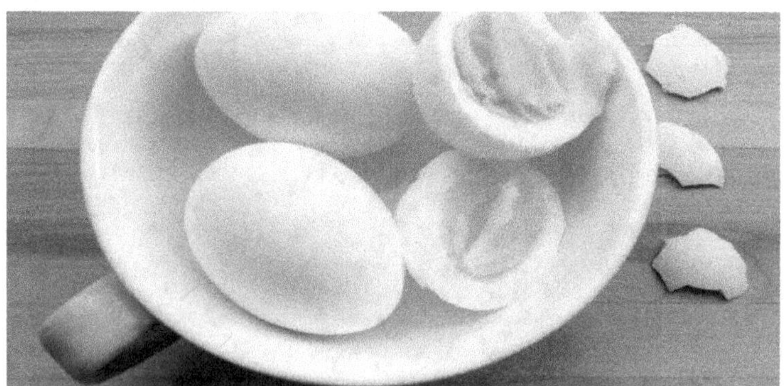

- Eggs: Eggs for nutritional needs in the third trimester

Eggs are an excellent source of choline, which aids in the normal functioning of cells and the fast growth of the fetus. Choline assists in memory development and minimizes the incidence of renal and pancreatic problems. You may eat a completely cooked egg in your breakfast.

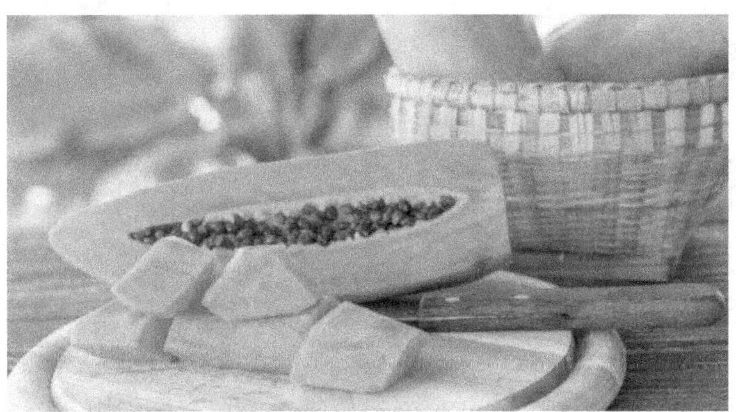

- Ripened papaya: It is an excellent source of vitamin C, fiber, potassium, and folate. It also aids in avoiding heartburns that are frequent during the third trimester. However, do not consume unripe papaya since it contains pepsin, which might promote contractions and early labor.

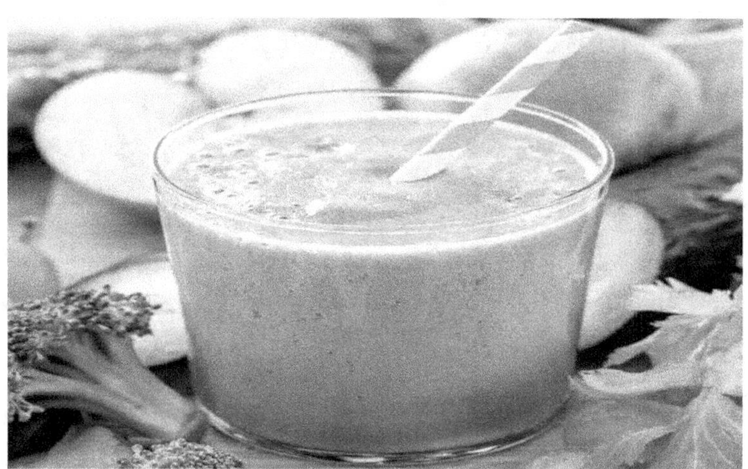

- Green smoothies: Green smoothies for nutritional needs in the third trimester

Green smoothies are a good source of fiber, calcium, vitamin B6, magnesium, and potassium. A mix of baby spinach or kale with ice creates an outstanding green smoothie. You may use coconut water and add additional ingredients like berries, pineapple, orange, mango, mint, or ginger to improve the flavor of the smoothie.

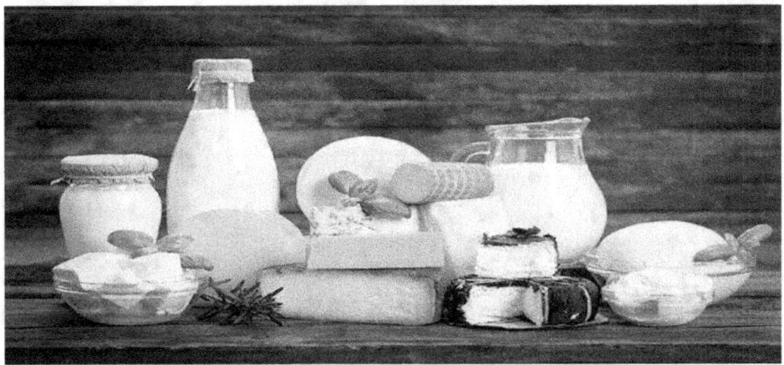

- Milk and milk products: Best milk and milk products for nutritional needs in the third trimester

These are excellent sources of calcium. By the third trimester, your calcium demand rises. Milk and milk products together with calcium supplements as suggested by the doctor can help you reach the need.

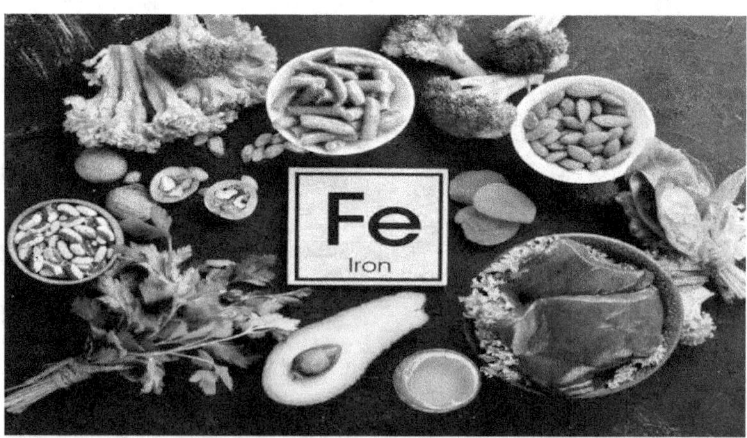

- Iron-rich meals: Iron-rich foods for nutritional needs in the third trimester

Green vegetables, broccoli, lean steak, and pork are high in iron. Iron is important for the increased flow of blood to the placenta during the third trimester.

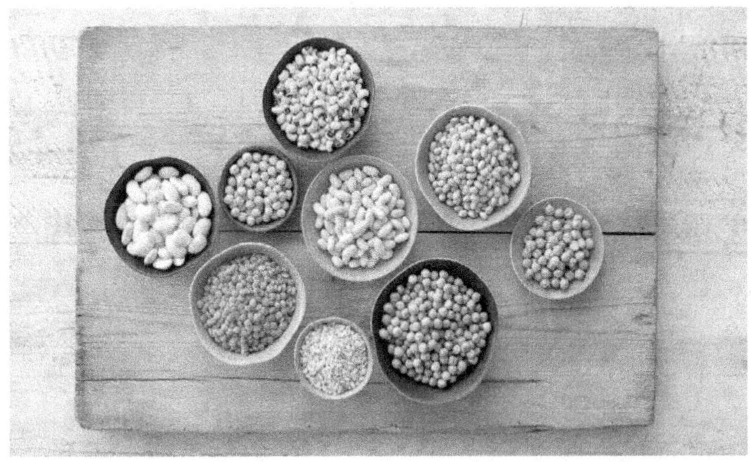

- Folic acid-rich diet: Folic acid diet for nutritional needs in the third trimester

Folic acid prevents neural tube abnormalities in the growing fetus. Bread, yeast, beans, chickpeas, and green leafy vegetables like spinach are also excellent sources of folic acid.

Now you know there is a large list of meals that you need to cover throughout the third trimester. It might be tough to remember and consume each item unless you have a strategy in place.

Useful Dietary Tips for Third Trimester

Here are some nutritional suggestions that you should follow throughout the third trimester of your pregnancy.

- Do not miss any meals and consume modest meals.
- Make sure your regular diet contains all food categories necessary.
- Cutaway sugar and salt-laden meals or snacks from your diet.
- Reduce the use of caffeinated drinks.
- Quit smoking
- Avoid eating fried and spicy meals since they might contribute to heartburn and indigestion.

A Sample Diet Plan for the Third Trimester of Pregnancy

Here is an example of a diet plan. You may follow this or adjust it to fit your needs in such a manner that you obtain the appropriate calories and all the vital elements.

	BREAKFAST	SNACK	LUNCH	SNACK	DINNER
Monday	Oats porridge with honey Apple juice	Sapodilla	Potato and onion paratha with curd, coriander and mint chutney	Mango panna and sprouted green gram chaat	Soya and mushroom curry and okra sabzi with cucumber and carrot salad+chapati/rice
Tuesday	Grilled paneer sandwich and Tea	Guava	Kidney beans curry + capsicum and cauliflower sabzi and cucumber raita+rice	Almond milk	Red lentil dal + beans sabzi + chapati/rice
Wednesday	Wheat porridge with dates and milk	Grapes	Potato and peas curry + pumpkin sabzi + chapati	Butter milk with dhokla	Spinach paratha + beetroot raita
Thursday	Sago upma with peanuts + coffee	Dried figs	Vegetable khichdi + pomegranate raita + roasted papad	Coconut water + roasted corn	Bottlegourd kofta curry + crispy lotus stem sabzi with Pearl millet roti
Friday	Semolina and mixed vegetable	Mango	Black gram dal + round gourd sabzi	Lassi + puffed rice with	Pulao with onion and tomato

	chila + buttermilk		and Chickpea flour + chapati	roasted peanuts	raita
Saturday	Methi paratha with curd	Papaya	Mung bean dal and carrot and peas with chapati/rice	Jal jeera + sweet potato chaat	Black-eyed peas curry + radish sabzi with roti
Sunday	Wholewheat toast with sautéed mushroom + banana milkshake	Pomegra nate	Chickpeas curry + bitter gourd sabzi with chapati/rice	Lemonade with + mixed nuts and raisins	Pasta in tomato sauce + steamed broccoli sticks

What to Avoid in the Third Trimester of Pregnancy

Avoid including these items in your third-trimester pregnant diet.

- Salt: Avoid consuming salty meals such as potato chips and fries.

- Raw Vegetables: Raw vegetables or uncooked veggies might lead to a gas issue, so you must avoid eating raw veggies. Before consuming any vegetable, make sure you cook it properly.

- Spicy Meals: Spicy foods may induce indigestion and heartburn during pregnancy, so they are best avoided in the latter trimester.

If a healthy diet has always been your philosophy, pregnant or not, you won't need to make any substantial adjustments. But if not, then make some dietary adjustments in the third trimester as well. You have done so well so far, so continue with that and your kid will develop appropriately! However, please consult with your doctor before incorporating anything into your diet, and enjoy a healthy pregnancy!

CHAPTER 4

FOODS AND BEVERAGES TO AVOID DURING PREGNANCY - WHAT NOT TO EAT

One of the first things individuals learn when they're pregnant is what they can't eat. It may be a huge letdown if you're major sushi, coffee, or rare steak aficionado.

Thankfully, there's more you can eat than you can't. You simply have to learn how to navigate the waters (the low mercury seas, that is) (the low mercury waters, that is).

You'll want to pay careful attention to what you eat and drink to be healthy.

Certain foods should only be taken seldom, while others should be avoided outright. Here are foods and drinks to avoid or reduce when pregnant.

1. High mercury fish

Mercury is a very hazardous element. It has no known safe amount of exposureTrusted Source and is most usually found in dirty water.

At greater levels, it may be hazardous to your brain system, immunological system, and kidneys. It may also cause major developmental issues in children, having detrimental consequences even at lesser levels.

Since it's present in dirty environments, huge marine fish may acquire enormous quantities of mercury. Therefore, it's advisable to avoid heavy mercury seafood when pregnant and nursing.

High-mercury fish you want to avoid include:

- Shark
- Swordfish
- King mackerel tuna (particularly bigeye tuna)
- Marlin
- Tilefish from the Gulf of Mexico
- Orange roughy

However, it's crucial to realize that not all fish are rich in mercury – only particular species.

Consuming low mercury fish during pregnancy is quite beneficial, and these fish may be eaten up to three times per week according to the Food and Drug Administration (FDA) (FDA).

Low mercury fish are numerous and include:

- Anchovies
- Cod
- Flounder
- Haddock
- Salmon

- Tilapia
- Trout (freshwater)

Fatty fish like salmon and anchovies are particularly ideal selections since they are rich in omega-3 fatty acids, which are necessary for your infant.

2. Undercooked or uncooked seafood

This one will be difficult for you sushi enthusiasts, but it's an essential one. Raw seafood, particularly shellfish, may cause various diseases. These may be viral, bacterial, or parasitic illnesses, such as norovirus, Vibrio, Salmonella, and Listeria.

Some of these illnesses may solely affect you, producing dehydration and weakness.

Other infections may be passed on to your kid with significant, or even deadly, effects.

Pregnant women are more prone to listeria infections. In fact, according to the Centers for Disease Control and Prevention (CDC), pregnant women are up to 10 times more likely to be infected with Listeria than the general population. Pregnant Hispanic women are 24 times more at risk.

This bacterium may be found in soil and polluted water or plants. Raw fish may get contaminated during processing, including smoking or drying.

Listeria bacteria may be transferred to your kid via the placenta, even if you're not displaying any symptoms of sickness. This may lead to preterm delivery, miscarriage, stillbirth, and other major health concerns, according to the CDC.

It's suggested to avoid raw fish and shellfish, including numerous sushi meals. But don't worry, you'll appreciate it that much more when the baby is delivered and it's safer to eat again.

3. Undercooked, uncooked, and processed meat

Some of the same risks with raw fish impact undercooked beef, too. Eating undercooked or raw meat raises your risk of illness from various bacteria or parasites, including Toxoplasma, E. coli, Listeria, and Salmonella.

Bacteria may jeopardize the health of your young one, perhaps leading to stillbirth or serious neurological diseases, including intellectual impairment, blindness, and epilepsy.

While most germs are found on the surface of complete chunks of meat, some bacteria may stay within the muscle fibers.

Some complete pieces of meat — such as tenderloins, sirloins, or ribeye from beef, lamb, and veal — may be safe to ingest when not cooked all the way through. However, this only applies when the piece of meat is entire or uncut, and thoroughly cooked on the exterior.

Cut meat, including beef patties, burgers, minced meat, pig, and chicken, should never be ingested uncooked or undercooked. So keep those burgers on the grill well done for now.

Hot dogs, lunch meat, and deli meat are also of concern, which is frequently shocking to pregnant individuals. These varieties of meat may get contaminated with different microorganisms during preparation or storage.

Pregnant women should not ingest processed meat items until they've been reheated to boiling.

4. Raw eggs

Raw eggs may be infected with the Salmonella bacterium.

Symptoms of salmonella infections include fever, nausea, vomiting, stomach cramps, and diarrhea.

In rare situations, the infection may induce uterine cramping, which can lead to preterm delivery or loss.

Foods that commonly contain raw eggs include:

- Lightly scrambled eggs
- Poached eggs
- Hollandaise sauce

- Homemade mayonnaise
- Some homemade salad dressings
- Homemade ice cream
- Homemade cake icings

Most commercial items containing raw eggs are manufactured with pasteurized eggs and are safe to ingest. However, you should always read the label to make sure.

To be on the safe side, always fully boil eggs or use pasteurized eggs. Save those super runny yolks and homemade mayo until after the baby makes its debut.

5. Organ meat

Organ meat has a wide range of nutrients.

These include iron, vitamin B12, vitamin A, zinc, selenium, and copper – all of which are excellent for you and your baby. However, taking too much animal-based vitamin A (preformed vitamin A) is not suggested during pregnancy.

Consuming too much-preformed vitamin A, particularly in the first trimester of pregnancy, may lead to congenital abnormalities and miscarriage.

Although this is usually related to vitamin A supplements, it's advisable to reduce your intake of organ meats like liver to just a few ounces once each week.

6. Caffeine

You may be one of the millions of persons who adore their daily cups of coffee, tea, soft drinks, or chocolate. You're not alone when it comes to our love of coffee.

Pregnant individuals are typically recommended to restrict their caffeine consumption to fewer than 200 milligrams (mg) per day, according to the American College of Obstetricians and Gynecologists (ACOG) (ACOG).

Caffeine is absorbed extremely fast and goes readily into the placenta. Because babies and their placentas don't have the main enzyme needed to metabolize caffeine, high levels can build up.

Caffeine use during pregnancy has been linked to fetal development restriction and an increased risk of low birth weight at delivery.

Low birth weight — less than 5 pounds, 8 ounces (or 2.5 kilograms) — is linked to an increased risk of newborn mortality and a greater risk of chronic disorders in adulthood.

So keep an eye on your daily cup of coffee or soda to ensure that your kid isn't getting too much caffeine.

7. Raw sprouts

Your healthy salad option may also include erroneous elements. Raw sprouts, including alfalfa, clover, radish, and mung bean sprouts, may be infected with Salmonella.

The humid climate needed for seeds to start sprouting is excellent for these sorts of bacteria, and they're virtually tough to wash off.

For this reason, you're recommended to avoid raw sprouts completely. However, sprouts are okay to ingest once they have been cooked, according to the FDA.

8. Unwashed produce

The surface of unwashed or unpeeled fruits and vegetables may be infected with numerous germs and parasites.

These include Toxoplasma, E. coli, Salmonella, and Listeria, which may be obtained through the soil or by handling.

Contamination may occur at any point during cultivation, harvest, processing, storage, transit, or sale. One hazardous parasite that may persist in fruits and vegetables is called Toxoplasma.

The majority of individuals who have toxoplasmosis have no symptoms, but some may feel like they have the flu for a month or longer.

Most children who are infected with the Toxoplasma bacterium while still in the womb show no symptoms at birth. However, symptoms such as blindness or intellectual problems may arise later in life.

What's more, a tiny fraction of infected babies suffers major eye or brain damage at birth.

While you're pregnant, it's extremely essential to decrease the danger of infection by carefully washing with water, and peeling, or boiling fruits and vegetables. Keep it up as a good habit once the baby comes, too.

9. Unpasteurized milk, cheese, and fruit juice

Raw milk, unpasteurized cheese, and soft-ripened cheeses may contain an assortment of hazardous bacteria, including Listeria, Salmonella, E. coli, and Campylobacter. (These are surely sounding familiar by now.)

The same applies to unpasteurized juice, which is also prone to bacterial infection. These illnesses may all have life-threatening effects on an unborn baby.

The bacteria might naturally exist or be induced by contamination during collection or storage. Pasteurization is the most effective way to kill any harmful bacteria, without changing the nutritional value of the products.

Consume only pasteurized milk, cheese, and fruit juice to reduce the chance of illness.

10. Alcohol

It is strongly suggested to avoid consuming alcohol while pregnant since it increases the chance of miscarriage and stillbirth. Even a small amount can negatively impact your baby's brain development.

Alcohol use during pregnancy may also result in fetal alcohol syndrome, a condition characterized by facial abnormalities, cardiac issues, and intellectual incapacity.

Because no dose of alcohol has been demonstrated to be safe during pregnancy, it is advised to avoid it entirely.

11. Processed junk foods

There's no better time than pregnancy to start eating nutrient-dense foods to help both you and your growing little one. You'll need larger quantities of numerous critical nutrients, including protein, folate, choline, and iron.

It's also a fallacy that you're "eating for two." You may eat as you typically do during the first semester, then increase by around 350 calories per day in your second trimester, and about 450 calories per day in your third trimester.

An optimum pregnant eating plan should mostly consist of complete foods, with sufficient nutrients to suit your and baby's requirements. Processed junk food is often poor in nutrition and heavy in calories, sugar, and added fats.

While some weight increase is required during pregnancy, excess weight gain has been related to several difficulties and disorders. These include a higher risk of gestational diabetes, as well as pregnancy or delivery problems.

Stick to meals and snacks that emphasize protein, vegetables, and fruits, healthy fats, and fiber-rich carbs like whole grains, beans, and starchy vegetables. Don't worry, there are tons of ways to sneak vegetables into your meals without compromising flavor.

In summary, while you're pregnant, it's crucial to avoid foods and drinks that may put you and your baby in danger.

Although most meals and drinks are completely fine to consume, others, including raw fish, unpasteurized dairy, alcohol, and high mercury seafood, should be avoided.

Plus, certain meals and drinks like coffee and foods rich in added sugar, should be reduced to support a healthy pregnancy.

Common Discomforts Of Pregnancy

You may be unpleasant at times throughout pregnancy. Discomforts like back ache and being tired are common and shouldn't make you worry.

For most discomforts, you can do numerous things to help you feel better.

Don't use any prescription, supplement, or herbal product to address pain without talking to your practitioner first. Some may harm your baby.

If any of the discomforts become severe or unpleasant or interfere with your normal life, inform your physician straight away.

Acne

What can I do about acne during pregnancy?

Acne may not cause you physical discomfort, but it may be annoying. If you've never had it, you may acquire it for the first time during pregnancy. If you've had it before pregnancy, it may get worse during pregnancy. We don't know precisely why acne develops during pregnancy, but it's probably due to additional hormones in your body.

To cure acne during pregnancy:

- Wash your face in the morning and night with a light cleanser and lukewarm water.

- If your hair is greasy, wash it with shampoo every day. Try to keep your hair off your face.

- Don't pick or squeeze acne. This may cause scarring.

- Use oil-free makeup. Look for the phrases water-based, noncomedogenic, or non-acnegenic on the product label.

- Talk to your health care practitioner about drugs you may take to treat acne. Don't take any medicine—even acne medicine—without talking to your physician beforehand. Some acne medications can be harmful to your baby. Some can cause birth defects.

Here's everything you need to know about acne medicine:

Most over-the-counter acne treatments are safe to take during pregnancy but check with your practitioner first. During pregnancy, you may be permitted to utilize goods that contain:

- Azelaic acid
- Glycolic acid
- Topical benzoyl peroxide
- Topical salicylic acid

Dapsone, a newer acne medication, may be safe to take during pregnancy, but check with your doctor first.

Some acne medications are not safe to take during pregnancy. They may create major complications for your kid, including birth abnormalities. Don't use these medicines during pregnancy:

- Hormonal therapy
- Isotretinoin and other retinoids
- Oral and topical tetracyclines

Talk to your provider before you take any medicine during pregnancy. Make sure any clinician you visit (such as a doctor who has particular expertise to treat skin, hair, and nails [dermatologist]) knows you're pregnant.

Back pain and sciatica

What can I do about back discomfort and sciatica during pregnancy?

Lower-back discomfort during pregnancy may be caused by pregnancy hormones, your increasing belly, and weight gain, particularly in the latter months. Pressure from the uterus may impact your sciatic nerve, which extends from the lower back to the hip and down the back of the leg. Pain along the sciatic nerve is termed sciatica.

Here's what you can do to help reduce back discomfort during pregnancy:

- Stand up straight with your chest high and your shoulders back and relaxed.

Don't lock your knees. Avoid standing for long periods. If you have to stand for a long period, attempt to rest one foot at a time on a stool or box.

- Sit on chairs that provide decent back support. Put a small pillow behind your lower back for extra support.

- Wear shoes with low heels and sufficient arch support. Don't wear flats or high heels. Don't lift heavy stuff. To pick up anything from the floor, bend at the knees and maintain your back straight. Don't sag around the waist.

- Sleep on your left side and put a pillow between your legs or sleep with a full body pillow. Use a firm mattress when sleeping. If your mattress is soft, put a board between it and the box spring to make it feel firmer.

- Wear maternity trousers with a broad elastic band that runs under your tummy. You may wish to consider wearing a belly-support girdle manufactured particularly for use during pregnancy.

- Aim to be active every day. Talk to your health care practitioner about exercises and stretches you may take to help strengthen your back muscles.

- Try placing a heating pad or ice pack on your back.

- Talk to your physician before you take any pain medication. This covers prescription and over-the-counter drugs, vitamins, and herbal products.

Call your provider straight away if:

- If your back pain is severe or if you also have a fever.
- Your feet feel numb or your legs are weak.
- You feel terrible discomfort in your calves.
- It burns when you pee (urinate) (urinate).
- You're bleeding from your vagina.

Belly ache

What can I do about discomfort in my lower belly?

As your baby develops, the muscles surrounding the uterus (womb) strain and stretch. This might cause soreness down in your tummy. You may feel it most when you cough or sneeze. It normally goes away if you keep motionless for a little or if you adjust to a different position.

Call your health care practitioner if your tummy discomfort is severe, becomes worse, or doesn't go away.

Breasts

What can I do about aching breasts during pregnancy?

Your breasts begin to alter early in pregnancy as they become prepared to generate breast milk to nourish your baby. Breast alterations include:

- Getting larger, fuller, and heavier. They may even look enlarged. Tender, swollen breasts may be one of the earliest indicators that you're pregnant. Your breasts enlarge due to pregnancy hormones and the development of fat and milk glands in them. As the skin on your breasts develops, it may be itchy and you may experience stretch marks.

- Nipples and areolas turning darker. Your nipples may jut out further, and the areolas may become bigger. The areola is the black region surrounding the nipple.

- Leaking colostrum. Colostrum is clear, sticky substance that comes out of your breasts shortly after delivery before your breast milk comes in. Your body begins manufacturing it during the final several months of pregnancy. As you come closer to your due date, colostrum may flow from your breasts.

Here's what you can do to assist reduce discomfort in your breasts:

- Get a decent maternity bra that has broad straps and wider cups.
- If you work out, be sure your bra provides you with adequate support.
- If your breasts itch, try the lotion. Talk to your health care professional about what type to use.

- If you are leaking colostrum, you may obtain pads to place in your bra cups to absorb the milk.

If the discomfort in your breasts doesn't go away, is severe or you notice a lump in your breast, notify your physician. If you've undergone breast surgery or implants, notify your physician.

Congestion and nosebleeds

What can I do about congestion and nosebleeds during pregnancy?

You may experience a runny or stuffy nose (nasal congestion) or nosebleeds during pregnancy. They're caused by increased pregnant hormones and blood in your body that makes the lining of your nose expand, dry up and bleed.

Here's what you can do if you have or want to avoid a stuffy or runny nose or nosebleed:

- Use a humidifier to enhance the moisture in the air in your house.
- Drink lots of water.
- Put a few dabs of petroleum jelly on the insides of your nose.
- Use saline nasal drops or nose rinse. Don't use any other form of drug without talking to your physician beforehand.

If you get a nosebleed:

- Sit up straight and lean forward.

- Breathe through your mouth and clamp your nose shut for 5 to 10 minutes with your thumb and finger.
- If you get blood in your mouth, spit it out. Swallowing it may upset your stomach.

Call your health care provider immediately away if:

- You have indicators of a cold or the flu, such as sneezing, coughing, a sore throat, fever, or mild pains.
- A nosebleed lasts more than 20 minutes.
- You develop a nosebleed following an injury to your head.

Constipation

What can I do about constipation during pregnancy?

Constipation is prevalent later in pregnancy. It's when you don't have bowel motions or they don't happen regularly, or your stools (poop) are hard to pass. Constipation during pregnancy may be caused by pregnancy hormones and the weight of your developing uterus, which may impair the process of how your body breaks down food after you eat (digestion) (digestion).

Here's what you can do to help treat constipation during pregnancy:

- Drink plenty of water. Fruit juice (particularly prune juice) may aid, too.

- Eat meals that are rich in fiber, such as fruits, vegetables, beans, whole-grain bread, and pasta and bran cereal.

- Eat smaller meals many times a day. Smaller quantities of food may be simpler to digest.

- Do something active every day. Walking is excellent. Ask your clinician about additional activities that are safe during pregnancy.

- Tell your provider about any supplements you take, particularly an iron supplement. Too much iron might contribute to constipation. Don't take any drug, supplement, or herbal product during pregnancy without talking to your physician beforehand. A supplement is a substance you take to make up for specific nutrients that you don't receive enough of in the meals you consume.

- Ask your clinician about over-the-counter medication that is safe to take. Don't take any form of medication during pregnancy without talking to your physician beforehand.

If you haven't had a bowel movement in 3 days, contact your physician straight away.

Fatigue and sleep issues

What can I do about exhaustion and sleep issues during pregnancy?

Fatigue is being exceedingly weary and having little energy. You may experience weariness early and late in pregnancy. Your body may feel fatigued because:

- It's working hard to take care of your developing kid. Your body's generating pregnant hormones and you're spending a lot of energy, even while you sleep.
- You may have difficulties sleeping at night because you're uncomfortable or you need to get up to go to the toilet. Later in pregnancy, leg cramps may keep you up at night.
- You may experience greater tension than before you were pregnant. Stress is a concern that you experience in

reaction to things that happen in your life. Stress might make you feel weary.

- You may have additional children to take care of and other activities that take up a lot of your time.

Here's what you can do to help you feel less tired:

- Try to go to bed and wake up at the same time every day. Take brief naps throughout the day, if you can.
- Eat healthful meals. Drink lots of water throughout the day but reduce it by a few hours before you go to bed at night.
- Every day, do something physical. Talk to your health care provider

about activities that are safe during pregnancy.

- Cut down on activities that aren't required or that make you sleepy. Ask your spouse, family, and friends to assist you out around the home or doing errands. If you have sick days or vacation days at work, utilize them.

Here's what you can do to help you get a decent night's sleep:

- Sleep on your left side with a pillow under your tummy and another one under your legs.
- Take a warm shower or bath before you go to bed to help you relax.
- Do activities, like yoga, to help you relax before going to bed.

- Make sure your bedroom is peaceful and pleasant.

- Cut off caffeine, particularly before sleep. Caffeine is a substance found in products like coffee, tea, soda, chocolate, and various energy drinks and pharmaceuticals. It stimulates the brain, therefore it makes you feel awake. It lingers in the body for many hours, so restrict it in the afternoon or evening.

Call your provider straight away if you're excessively exhausted or if it starts to interfere with your regular life.

Gas

What can I do to help minimize gas during pregnancy?

During pregnancy, various hormones and your developing baby crowding your belly might slow down the process of how your body breaks down food after you eat (digestion) and cause you to bloat, burp, and release gas.

Here's what you can do to help minimize gas during pregnancy:

- Don't consume foods that induce gas, such as fried or greasy meals, beans, cabbage, cauliflower, and dairy products, like milk and cheese. Limit meals and beverages that are carbonated (bubbly), like soda.

- Eat numerous little meals throughout the day.
- Do something active every day. Exercise may assist improve digestion. Talk to your clinician about safe things to undertake during pregnancy.
- Talk to your health care practitioner before you use any medication to assist alleviate gas and bloating.

Call your provider straight away if you have:

- Gas that feels like labor contractions, that comes and goes frequently, every 5-10 minutes. Contractions happen when the muscles of your uterus go tense and then release. Contractions assist push your baby out of your uterus.

- Blood in your stool (poop) (poop)
- Severe diarrhea
- Nausea (feeling ill to your stomach) and vomiting.

Headaches

What can I do to help alleviate headaches during pregnancy?

Headaches are typical during pregnancy, particularly in the first trimester. They're generally triggered by pregnancy hormones, stress, or physical strain caused by carrying additional weight during pregnancy. If you're cutting down on caffeine during pregnancy, you may have a headache until your body gets acclimated to the new level.

Here's what you can do to help reduce headaches during pregnancy:

- Talk to your health care practitioner before you use any drug, supplement, or natural product to ease your headache. Some may be dangerous to your infant. A supplement is a substance you take to make up for specific nutrients that you don't receive enough of in the meals you consume. An herbal product, such as a pill or tea, is created from herbs (plants) that are used in cooking.
- Try to discover what triggers your headache (called a headache trigger)

(called a headache trigger). Common headache causes include cigarette smoke, certain meals, and eye strain. Once you know your triggers, strive to reduce or get rid of them.

- Eat nutritious meals, drink plenty of water and do something active every day.

- Get a good night's sleep every night. Rest throughout the day when you can.

- Try to lessen your stress. Stress is concern, strain, or pressure that you experience in reaction to things that happen in your life. Tell your health care physician if you need support to lower your stress.

- Try relaxing methods, such as deep breathing, yoga, and massage. Take a warm shower or bath before you go to bed.

- Put a moist towel on your head or the back of your neck.

Call your provider straight away if your headache:

- Is harsh or doesn't go away? Severe headaches during pregnancy may be an indication of preeclampsia. This disorder may arise after the 20th week of pregnancy. It's when a woman has high blood pressure and indicators like a strong headache that signal that some of her organs aren't performing correctly.
- Comes with fever, visual abnormalities, slurred speech,

tiredness, numbness or not being able to keep attentive.

- Comes after falling or striking your head.
- Comes with a stuffy nose, headache, pressure beneath your eyes, or a toothache. These may be indicators of a sinus infection.

Heartburn

What can I do to help alleviate heartburn during pregnancy?

Heartburn is a painful, burning sensation in the throat or chest. It occurs when food or stomach acid backs up into the tube that delivers food, drink, and saliva from your mouth to your stomach (esophagus)

(esophagus). Heartburn is frequent during pregnancy because pregnancy hormones loosen the valve between the stomach and the esophagus, and your developing uterus (womb) increases pressure on your stomach.

Here's what you can do to help reduce heartburn during pregnancy:

- Eat five or six modest meals a day instead of three big ones. Eat meals slowly—don't hurry.
- Drink more fluids between meals and less with meals.
- Don't eat late at night. Eat your final meal two to three hours before you lay down or go to bed.

- Don't consume things that trigger heartburn, such as greasy or fatty meals, spicy foods, citrus goods (like oranges or orange juice), and chocolate.
- Don't consume alcohol. Drinking alcohol during pregnancy might create major difficulties for your kid.
- Raise your head on pillows while you sleep.
- Talk to your health care practitioner before you take any drug, such as an antacid, to assist alleviate heartburn.

Call your provider straight away if you:

- Have heartburn that returns as soon as your antacid wears off.

- Have heartburn that keeps you up at night.
- Have difficulties swallowing.
- Are spitting up blood and have black stools (poop).
- Are losing weight.

Hemorrhoids

What can I do to treat hemorrhoids during pregnancy?

Hemorrhoids are bulging veins in and around the place where excrement exits the body (rectum) (rectum). They're itchy and painful. During pregnancy, they're caused by increased blood flow in the pelvic region and the strain on veins there from your developing uterus. Constipation might make them worse. Constipation is when you don't have bowel motions or they don't happen regularly, or your stools (poop) are hard to pass.

Here's what you can do to help avoid hemorrhoids during pregnancy:

- Eat meals that are rich in fiber, such as fruit, vegetables, beans, whole-grain bread and pasta, and bran cereal.
- Drink lots of water.
- Do something active every day. Talk to your health care provider about activities that are safe during pregnancy.
- Gain the proper amount of weight throughout pregnancy. Talk to your

physician about how much you should gain.

- Try not to push too hard when you poop.

Here's what you can do to assist treat hemorrhoids during pregnancy:

- Don't sit for lengthy periods. Get up and walk around to help take the weight of your uterus off of the pelvic veins.

- Soak in a warm tub a couple of times each day. Make sure the water isn't hot.

- Ask your physician about over-the-counter medication (creams or wipes) that are safe to use during pregnancy. Also, enquire about fiber supplements and stool (poop) softeners. Don't take any drug, supplement, or herbal product without talking to your physician first. Over-the-counter medication is the medicine you may acquire without a prescription from your physician. A supplement is a substance you take to make up for specific nutrients that you don't receive enough of in the meals you consume. An herbal product, such as a pill or tea, is created from herbs (plants) that are used in cooking.

- Talk to your physician about using an ice patch or witch hazel pads to assist alleviate discomfort and swelling.

If you experience bleeding or severe discomfort, contact your physician straight away.

Leg cramps

What can I do to ease leg cramps during pregnancy?

Leg cramps in your lower legs (calves) and even in your feet are prevalent in the second and third trimesters. They commonly happen at night and might wake you awake. We're not precisely clear what causes leg cramps in pregnancy.

Here's what you can do to help avoid leg cramps:

- Stretch your legs before you go to bed.

- Do something active every day. Talk to your health care physician about activities that are safe to undertake during pregnancy.

- Eat meals that are rich in magnesium. Magnesium is a mineral that you receive through diet. Too little magnesium in your body may induce leg cramps. Foods that contain a lot of magnesium in them include whole-grain bread and pasta, beans, nuts, seeds, and dried fruit. Ask your physician about taking a magnesium supplement. A supplement is a merchandise you take to make up for specific nutrients that you don't receive enough of in meals you consume.

- Drink plenty of water.
- Wear comfy and supportive shoes.
- Talk to your doctor about taking a calcium supplement.

Here's what you can do to assist cure leg cramps:

- Stretch your calf muscles. Flex your feet and down.
- Massage the calves with long, downward strokes.
- Take a hot shower or a heated bath.
- Put ice on your legs.

Call your provider if your leg cramps:

- Happen a lot
- Causes significant agony

- Come with edema, redness, skin changes, or weak muscles
- Don't get better when you attempt to alleviate them.

Shortness of breath

What can I do to assist with shortness of breath during pregnancy?

Shortness of breath occurs when you do not feel as if you are getting enough air into your lungs when you breathe. You may feel like this later in pregnancy when your baby's huge and pulling on the muscle that helps you breathe (diaphragm) (diaphragm). Even if you sense shortness of breath, your baby's receiving oxygen in the womb.

To assist make breathing easier:

- Don't smoke. If you need support to stop smoking, inform your health care practitioner.
- Sit or stand up straight to allow your lungs space to expand. Move gently.
- Try to breathe pure air. Stay away from secondhand smoke (smoke from someone else's cigarettes) and other air contaminants.

Call your provider if:

- There's a dramatic shift in your respiration.
- You have a cough.
- You feel an ache in your chest.

Teeth and gums

How do teeth and gums alter during pregnancy?

You may not anticipate it, but your teeth and gums may alter during pregnancy. It's crucial to maintain your teeth and gums healthy so they don't become infected. Infections during pregnancy may create complications for you and your babies, such as raising your risk for preterm labor and early delivery. Preterm labor is labor that occurs before 37 weeks of pregnancy. Premature birth is a birth that occurred before 37 weeks of pregnancy.

Common dental and gum alterations include:

- Your gums may be sore and swollen. They may bleed when you brush or floss.
- Your teeth may feel loose. This may happen because pregnancy hormones that assist relax muscles for labor and delivery may loosen the tissue that keeps your teeth in place.
- If you suffer morning sickness, the acid in your mouth may cause the enamel on your teeth to wear off (erode) (erode). The acid also may create cavities.

Here's what you can do to assist ease any discomfort that may occur with tooth and gum changes:

- Use a softer toothbrush.
- Warm salt water should be used to rinse your mouth.
- Get regular dental checkups even during pregnancy. Make sure your dentist knows that you're pregnant.

Urinating frequently

What can I do about needing to urinate regularly during pregnancy?

You may need to pee (urinate) more regularly throughout pregnancy, particularly early in pregnancy and in the last weeks before your baby is due. As your baby develops, the weight pulls down on your bladder. Urine may flow when you cough, laugh, sneeze or exercise.

Here's what you can do if you need to urinate often:

- Don't consume coffee, tea, soda, and other liquids that contain caffeine in them. Caffeine is a medicine that might cause you to need to urinate more regularly.
- Do Kegel exercises to help strengthen the muscles that regulate the flow of urine. To perform these, squeeze the muscles you employ to stop yourself from urinating. Hold the muscles tight for 3 seconds and then relax. Do this 10 to 15 times, three times each day.

Kegel exercises can assist prepare muscles for labor and delivery.

- Go when you need to go. Don't attempt to hold it. When you urinate, bend forward a little to thoroughly empty your bladder.
- Go to the restroom before your workout. Talk to your health care provider about safe workouts to undertake during pregnancy.
- Stop consuming fluids for around 2 to 3 hours before you go to bed.
- Use a cushion or panty liner to collect leaks.

Call your physician immediately away if you develop signs or symptoms of a urinary tract infection (commonly called a UTI). If it's not treated, a UTI may lead to a more severe infection or premature delivery. Preterm labor is labor that occurs too soon, before 37 weeks of pregnancy. Signs and symptoms of UTIs include:

- Blood in the urine
- Fever
- Needing to go again quickly after you urinate
- Pain or burning when you urinate

Vaginal discharge

What do I need to know about vaginal discharge during pregnancy?

Vaginal discharge (commonly termed lochia) that's clear, white, or sticky is typical throughout pregnancy. It's caused by pregnancy-related changes in the birth canal (vagina) and the entrance to the uterus at the top of the vagina (cervix) (cervix).

Discharge that's not typical may be an indication of infection, and infections may cause major issues during pregnancy. Call your health care physician immediately away if you discharge:

- Is not clear or white
- Smells terrible
- Comes with itchiness
- Comes with discomfort or soreness

Varicose veins and swelling in your legs, ankles, and feet

What can I do about varicose veins and edema in my legs, ankles, and feet?

If you glance down and can't see your ankles, you're not alone! Many women develop swelling in their legs, ankles, and feet during pregnancy. Swelling may be caused by pregnancy hormones, having extra fluid in your body during pregnancy, and pressure from your developing baby on the veins that transport blood to your heart.

Pressure on a vein called the inferior vena cava may create uncomfortable, itchy, blue bulges on your legs. These are termed varicose veins. They normally don't create issues, but they're not beautiful. You're more likely to have them if it's your first pregnancy or if other individuals in your family have them.

Here's what you can do to help reduce varicose veins and swelling in your legs, ankles, and feet:

- Don't stand for lengthy periods.
- When you're sitting down, put your feet up. Don't cross your legs while you sit.
- When you're laying down, put your legs up on a pillow.
- Sleep on your left side. This removes strain off the vein that sends blood from the lower sections of your body to your heart.

- Wear support hose or compression stockings or leggings. These fit firmly all over and may help minimize edema. Don't wear socks or stockings that have a tight ring of elastic around the leg.
- Do something active every day. Talk to your physician about activities that are safe during pregnancy.
- Put an ice pack on swollen regions.

If you experience significant or abrupt swelling, notify your physician straight away. These may be indicators of a dangerous illness called preeclampsia. This disorder may arise after the twentieth week of pregnancy. It's when a woman has high blood pressure and indicators like a strong headache that signal that some of her organs aren't performing correctly.

CHAPTER 5

HERBAL MEDICINE USAGE DURING PREGNANCY

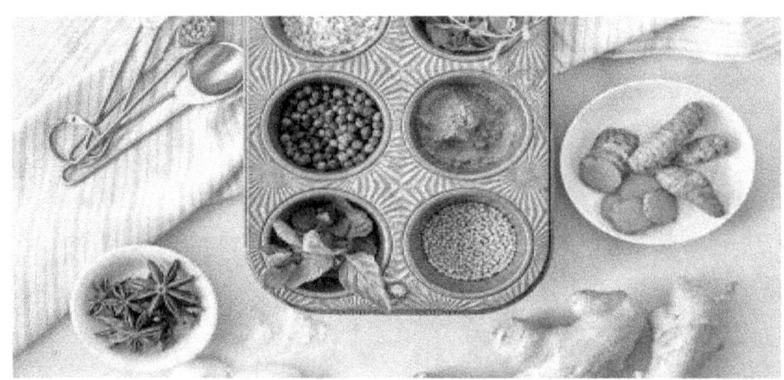

Herbal medicine has been utilized for illness prevention and treating disorders globally. It is known that between 65 and 85% of the global population utilized herbal medicine as their major source of health treatment.

The incidence of herbal medication usage during pregnancy varies from 12 to 82.3%. Ginger, garlic, raspberry, cranberry, valerian, chamomile, peppermint, and fenugreek are often used herbal medications during pregnancy. Using herbal medication during pregnancy has debatable difficulties. Even though herbal medication is freely accessible as compared to conventional drugs, the safety problem during pregnancy is a worry. Using herbal medication in the first 3 months and late in the third trimester is hazardous for the fetus.

Before taking any herbal treatment, it is important to visit the doctor and the pharmacist to confirm that the herbs are acceptable and safe to use during pregnancy. In pregnancy, moms are worried about any drugs that may impact their health, the health of the baby, and the pregnancy outcomes. Availing evidence-based knowledge on the advantages and unpleasant effects of herbal medicine usage during pregnancy is vital for a safer pregnancy and healthy baby.

Advantages and adverse consequences of Herbal medicine usage during pregnancy

Herbal medicine usage during pregnancy is ubiquitous throughout regions and nations. The incidence of herbal medicine usage during pregnancy varies vary between areas and nations. Multinational research done in several countries indicated that 28.9% of pregnant women utilized herbal medicine during pregnancy. A literature analysis from the Middle East indicated that up to 82.2% of the women utilized herbal medication at some time during pregnancy. The survey also found that many women utilized herbal medication throughout the first trimester. Observational cohort research done in South West England indicated that 26.7% of the women used a complementary or alternative medication at least once during pregnancy.

The usage of herbs grew from 6% in the first trimester to 12.4% in the second trimester and 26.3% in the third trimester. In Australia, 36% of the women used at least one herbal treatment during pregnancy. Studies done in Africa indicated the incidence of herbal medicine usage during pregnancy was between 12 to 73.1%.

The most widely taken herbal medications during pregnancy are; ginger, cranberry, valerian, raspberry leaf, chamomile, peppermint, rosehip, thyme, fenugreek, green tea, sage, and aniseed. Eucalyptus, tenaadam (Ruta chalepensis), damakess (Ocimum lamiifolium), feto, omore are some additional herbal treatments utilized during pregnancy, Garlic, palm kernel oil, bitter kola, and Dogon Yaro (Azadirachta indica) are some herbs that are utilized during pregnancy.

Being students, having no education, having a poor income, and having a tertiary education level made women more likely to take herbal medicine during pregnancy. The other criteria that make women more inclined to ingest herbal medications include being primiparas, non-smoking, and senior-age women.

Based on the existing investigations and literature reviews, the most often utilized herbal drugs during pregnancy are identified. The advantages and undesirable effects of the plants are also examined.

1. Ginger (Zingiber officinale)

Common names of ginger include African ginger, black ginger, Cochin ginger, gingembre, ginger root, imber, and Jamaica ginger.

Benefits of ginger

Ginger is used as an anti-nauseant and anti-emetic for nausea and hyperemesis gravidarum. The recommended daily intake of ginger is up to 1g of dry powder. A single-blind scientific experiment proved ginger as an effective herbal remedy for lowering nausea and vomiting during pregnancy. This research also indicated a daily total of 100 mg of ginger in a pill.

A randomized controlled clinical research done on 120 women over 20 weeks of gestation with symptoms of morning sickness demonstrated ingestion of 1500 mg of dried ginger for 4 days improved nausea and vomiting. The research also indicated that neonates whose moms took ginger during pregnancy had normal birth weights and normal APGAR scores. Consumption of ginger in proportions used in food preparation is believed to be safe. Taking 1–2 g of dried ginger for a day has been demonstrated to ease symptoms of the mild disorder of pregnancy. Using larger amounts of ginger is not safe for pregnant women. Thus, pregnant women should not consume a greater dosage of ginger.

Untoward effects of ginger

A literature study showed that ginger is not a safe herb. It is a possible abortifacient at large dosages (>1000 mg daily ingestion). Higher amounts of ginger might induce thinning of blood, stomach pain, and heartburn.

2. Garlic (Allium sativa)

Garlic is a perennial plant grown in several nations. It is extensively used as a cooking component and as a spice in many nations.

Benefits of garlic

A study done on the antimicrobial and antifungal activity of garlic indicated antibacterial and antifungal characteristics of garlic make it beneficial to ingest during pregnancy. Garlic increases a woman's immune system; this in turn assists women to have healthy pregnancies and healthy kids. Eating garlic during pregnancy is helpful to minimize the incidence of preeclampsia and protein retention in urine.

A randomized controlled trial was undertaken where 100 primigravidas were given either garlic tablets (800 mg/day) or placebo throughout the third trimester of pregnancy to investigate the impact of garlic tablet supplementation on preeclampsia. Except for a garlic aroma, minor negative effects like nausea were recorded due to garlic eating throughout the third trimester of pregnancy. Pregnancy outcomes were similar in both treatment with garlic and the placebo group. The research did not report any incidence of significant or minor abnormalities in newborn newborns and there were no spontaneous miscarriages of the fetuses.

Untoward effects of garlic

Excessive usage of garlic should be avoided in early pregnancy. Pregnant women with thyroid issues should avoid its usage. Pregnant women should also avoid taking garlic prior to surgery including cesarean as it may interfere with blood clotting. Another unpleasant consequence of taking garlic during pregnancy is that it may increase heartburn.

3. Cranberry (Vaccinium macrocarpon)

There are many sorts of cranberries: American cranberry, Arandano Americano, Arandano Trepador, Cranberries, European cranberry, Grosse Moosbeere, kranbeere, huge cranberry, Moosebeere, Mossberry.

Benefits of cranberry

Using cranberry during pregnancy is beneficial to avoid urinary tract infections, stomach ulcers, periodontal problems, and influenza. A study done on 400 Norwegian postpartum mothers found that cranberry was one of the most regularly utilized herbs after pregnancy, primarily for urinary tract infections.

Untoward effects of cranberries

The unfavorable consequences of cranberry usage during pregnancy warrants additional study.

4. Valerian (Valeriana officinalis)

Valerian is native to Europe and Asia and has naturalized in Eastern North America. It has been widely grown throughout Northern Europe.

Benefits of valerian

Valerian is used as a moderate sedative to assist patients to fall asleep and ease tension and anxiety. There is a dearth of safety information regarding the ingestion of valerian during pregnancy. It is strongly suggested that pregnant women consult with the doctor before consuming valerian during pregnancy. A study was done on the influence of valerian intake during pregnancy on cortical volume and the levels of zinc and copper in brain tissue of mouse fetuses indicating valerian consumption in pregnancy had no significant effect on brain weight and cerebral cortex volume and copper level in the fetal brain.

Untoward effects of valerian

Studies done on mouse fetuses demonstrated that the use of valerian during pregnancy had a considerable reduction in the amount of zinc in the brain. This data shows that valerian usage during pregnancy should be minimized.

5. Bitter kola

Bitter kola is a plant that originates from Africa. Africans have been utilizing bitter kola for pregnant women for centuries. Nowadays, bitter kola popularity has extended internationally.

Benefits of bitter kola

Drinking bitter kola is healthy during pregnancy. Bitter kola includes minerals and vitamins helpful for pregnancy. For Africans, bitter kola is the greatest compliment for pregnant women. Health advantages of bitter kola include relieving nausea and vomiting, making the uterus healthier, strengthening pregnant women, and restoring blood circulation in pregnant women. Bitter kola has extremely powerful caffeine. One bean of bitter kola has the same amount of caffeine as two cups of coffee. Thus, pregnant women have to drink the prescribed dosage (one small cup of bitter kola in a day) (one small cup of bitter kola in a day).

Untoward effects of bitter kola

Using very high doses of bitter kola is not recommended. A very high dosage of bitter kola is not beneficial for the uterus of the lady.

6.   Fenugreek   (Trigonella foenum-graecum)

Fenugreek is an annual leguminous herb that belongs to the family Fabaceae, which is found as a wild plant and farmed in Northern India. It is a galactagogue.

Benefits of fenugreek

Consumption of fenugreek during pregnancy boosts milk output in pregnant women. The precise mechanism of fenugreek ingestion and enhancing milk production is not fully known. However, it is thought that seeds of fenugreek contain the precursor of a hormone that promotes milk production.

Untoward effect of fenugreek

Large quantities of fenugreek may induce uterine contractions, miscarriage, or early labor. It might influence blood sugar levels, thus pregnant women with insulin-dependent diabetes mellitus should avoid it. It may also induce heartburn.

7. Red raspberry leaf (Rubus idaeus)

The red raspberry leaf is known as a garden raspberry leaf. The deciduous raspberry plant generates it.

Benefits of red raspberry

Red raspberry leaf is a mineral-rich nutritive and uterine tonic to encourage expedient labor with less hemorrhage. It may also be used as an astringent for diarrhea. In research based on two clinical trials, there was a favorable connection between red raspberry usage and astringency in the event of diarrhea. The Daily suggested dosage is 1.5–5g.

Traditionally, red raspberry leaf has been used in late pregnancy to decrease the time of labor and to minimize problems of pregnancy. Pregnant women should visit a doctor or a pharmacist for guidance before taking red raspberry leaf in pregnancy in a tea or infusion. Red raspberry fruit is not regarded to offer harm to the mother or the baby during pregnancy.

Some women take it as a labor assist during the final 2 months before birth, but others take it throughout the pregnancy. In a randomized clinical experiment, 192 women at 32 weeks of gestation got 1.2 g of raspberry leaf pills twice a day. The research found no detrimental effects on mothers or babies. The active therapy with raspberry leaf reduced the second stage of labor and decreased the rate of forceps delivery.

A retrospective observational research done on 108 pregnant women indicated that 57 women who swallowed raspberry leaves were less likely to have an artificial rupture of membranes or to need a cesarean section, forceps, or vacuum delivery than 51 controls. Women have used red raspberry leaves for uncomfortable times of pregnancy, and morning sickness, to avoid miscarriage, ease labor and delivery, and enrich breast milk.

Untoward effects of red raspberry

The unfavorable impact of red raspberry warrants additional study.

8. Chamomile (Matricaria recutita)

There are two varieties of chamomile: German and Roman. The popular German variant originates from the flower Matricaria recutita, while the less frequent Roman variation derives from the bloom Chamaemelum mobile. German chamomile is used in drinks and various supplements such as pills and oils.

Benefits of chamomile

Chamomile is used as a moderate sedative and to help digestion. It has been used for the treatment of morning sickness. German chamomile is the variety used most commonly as a medical plant, extracts of which have been found to enhance the tone of the uterine muscle.

Chamomile does not contain caffeine, which makes it safer for pregnant women, however, there is some disagreement regarding the safety of specific plants not completely specified by the Food and Drug Administration.

There is insufficient research to establish for sure if chamomile may cause damage during pregnancy. As with many other plants, the entire impact of chamomile, particularly in interaction with other drugs and herbs, has not been investigated satisfactorily.

Untoward effect of chamomile

Chamomile may induce increased blood flow, contractions, miscarriage, or preterm labor. It may also trigger adverse responses.

9. Clary sage (Salvia officinale)

Clary sage is a shrub native to Italy, Syria, and Southern France and thrives on dry soil. The essential oil is distilled from the flowers and blooming tips.

Benefits of clary sage

It is suggested that clary sage only be taken from 37 weeks onwards. It may be used to induce labor if the body is ready to go into labor. It may stimulate the release of oxytocin in pregnant women. Using clary sage is highly advised during labor to aid contractions to increase and become more effective in drawing up the horizontal uterine muscles to open the cervix and send the baby down into the pelvis and the birth canal.

The easiest and most frequent approach to utilize clary sage during labor is to place a few drops on to dry cloth; the mother will inhale the scent when she needs it to help herself feel more calm and relaxed during contractions.

Untoward effects of clary sage

Large dosages are best avoided for the risk of probable miscarriage and abortifacient impact.

10. Anise (Pimpinella anisum)

Anise is sometimes referred to as aniseed. There are two kinds of anise: anise (Pimpinella anisum) and star anise (Illicium verum) Chinese star anise.

Benefits of anise

Orally, anise is used for dyspepsia, flatulence, rhinorrhoea (runny nose), and as an expectorant, diuretic, and appetite stimulant. Anise is also used to enhance lactation and assist delivery. Topically, anise is utilized for lice, scabies, and psoriasis therapy. Using anise during pregnancy is generally safe when taken orally in doses usually seen in meals.

There is little trustworthy evidence available concerning the safety of anise when taken orally in medical dosages during pregnancy. Anise used in little doses in herbal tea is safer in pregnancy since exposure is very low.

Untoward effects of anise

When administered topically, anise in conjunction with other plants might induce localized pruritis. In allergic people, inhaled or swallowed anise may induce rhino conjunctivitis, occupational asthma, and anaphylaxis. Essential oil and concentrated anise should be avoided in pregnancy for the worry that they can cause early labor.

11. Green tea (Camellia sinensis)

Green tea is mainly eaten in the Middle East.

Benefits of green tea

Green tea is useful to control blood sugar, cholesterol, and blood pressure levels. It also boosts the body's metabolic rate and offers a natural source of energy. It may help regulate a pregnant mother's mood. However, taking too high a dosage of green tea is not suggested. The recommended dosage of caffeine per day is 300 mg.

Untoward effects of green tea

Pregnant women who drink green tea are at risk of spontaneous abortion as indicated by the following two studies. Case-control research done on 3149 pregnant women indicated that serum paraxanthine (caffeine metabolite) was greater in women who had spontaneous abortions than in controls.

Another case-control research done on 1498 pregnant women likewise revealed that the use of 375 mg or more caffeine per day during pregnancy can increase the chance of spontaneous abortion. Pregnant women who ingested excessive caffeine throughout pregnancy had a probability to produce low birth weight babies. This is corroborated by the following investigations. Prospective research done on 2291 pregnant women found that women who ingested more than 600 mg of caffeine per day are at increased risk for having low birth weight babies.

Prospective research is done on 63 women also found that pregnant women who took more than 300 mg/day of caffeine had low birth weight babies. Studies indicated ingestion of high levels of caffeine has an elevated risk of stillbirth. A prospective follow-up study on 18,478 singleton pregnancies found that the drinking of eight or more cups of coffee in a day quadrupled the chance of experiencing stillbirth compared with women who did not consume coffee.

Even though the aforementioned research is done on coffee intake, consumption of large dosages of green tea might have detrimental effects on mothers and their babies. The caffeine present in coffee and green tea is not significantly different.

Consumption of too much caffeine (more than 300 mg per day or more than eight cups per day) might induce miscarriage as evidenced by the following study results. Consumption of too much coffee might also create the problem of sleeping.

12. Thyme (Thymus vulgaris)

It is known as common thyme, French thyme, garden thyme, oil thyme, red thyme oil, rubbed thyme, Spanish thyme, thyme aetheroleum, thyme essential oil, thyme oil, thyme herbal, van ajwain, Vanya yavani, white thyme oil.

Benefits of thyme

A literature analysis done on herbal medicine usage during pregnancy found thyme is utilized to alleviate bloating and stomach discomfort. It is also used for the treatment of common colds and urinary tract infections.

When used in proportions usually seen in food, thyme has a generally recognized safe status in the US. There is inadequate trustworthy evidence available on the safety of thyme when taken at medical levels during pregnancy. Therefore, pregnant women should avoid consuming thyme in medication dosage.

Untoward effects of thyme

Consumption of a significant dosage of thyme produces an emmenagogue effect. Therefore, it is best to avoid it, particularly in early pregnancy, because of the risk of probable miscarriage.

13. Coconut

Countries within the Southeast Asian area are rich in coconut oil and other coconut by-products.

Benefits of coconut

Studies indicated that coconut oil has been utilized to assist labor, and delivery, and to avoid congenital deformity. Coconut oil during pregnancy may be utilized as a part of a balanced nutrient-dense whole food diet.

Coconut oil contains substantial levels of saturated fat with high concentrations of lauric acid. The saturated fat level helps to build up enough fat reserves in pregnancy and preparation for breastfeeding.

Untoward effects of coconut

The research undertaken to evaluate the impact of virgin coconut oil on mice demonstrated that virgin coconut oil might alter newborn development and appearance through maternal consumption. The research also urges the use of virgin coconut oil as herbal medicine must be addressed with care.

14. Echinacea (Echinacea spp)

Echinacea species come from North America and were historically utilized by the Indians for a range of illnesses, including mouth sores, colds, bruises, tooth discomfort, and bug bites.

Benefits of Echinacea

One clinical trial research demonstrates a favorable connection between echinacea intake in lowering duration and recurrence of cold and urinary tract infections. The suggested dosage is 5–20 ml tincture.

Untoward effects of Echinacea

The unfavorable impact of taking echinacea during pregnancy requires additional investigation.

15. Peppermint (Mentha piperita)

Peppermint is one of the world's oldest medicinal plants and is utilized in both Eastern and Western cultures. Ancient Greek, Roman, and Egyptian societies employed plants for food and medicinal. Peppermint is presently one of the most commercially significant aromatic and therapeutic crops produced in the US.

Benefits of peppermint

Several clinical investigations have demonstrated that peppermint essential oil, a very concentrated form of herbs, may help ease irritable bowel syndrome. Natural medicine's extensive database reveals there are no instances in the scientific literature of peppermint being either safe or contraindicated during pregnancy.

Peppermint leaves and oil are regarded to be safe during pregnancy when ingested in meal proportions. A study done on the usage of antiemetic herbs in pregnancy found that peppermint is utilized for the treatment of pregnancy-induced nausea.

Untoward effects of peppermint

The unfavorable impact of peppermint ingestion during pregnancy deserves additional research.

Herbs that are not safe during pregnancy

Some herbs are dangerous during pregnancy since they could induce preterm labor or other issues. Herbs to avoid during pregnancy include:

- Uterine stimulants like aloe, barberry, black cohosh, blue cohosh, dong Quai, feverfew, goldenseal, juniper, wild yam, and motherwort

- Herbs that can hurt your kid, such as autumn crocus, mugwort (acceptable for moxibustion but not for ingestion), pokeroot, and sassafras
- Herbs that have additional harmful effects, such as comfrey and mistletoe

Again, always talk with your health care professional before taking any herbal medicine and verify whether it's healthy for you and your baby.

CHAPTER 6

WHAT TO EAT WHILE BREASTFEEDING

You've heard that nursing is very good for your kid, but did you realize that breastfeeding provides advantages for your health as well?

Breastfeeding may help lower your chance of acquiring some medical disorders later in life, including heart disease and diabetes. It may also ease stress and help you feel more connected to your new baby. All excellent stuff.

Plus, breast milk is chock-full of nutritious nutrients and protecting chemicals that are vital for your baby's growth. This is why breast milk is considered the "gold standard" for newborn nourishment and is sometimes referred to as liquid gold.*

Add "producing liquid gold" to the long list of incredible things women are capable of achieving.

Not surprisingly, it takes a lot of energy to make this liquid gold, and your requirements for numerous nutrients grow to satisfy these demands.

It's so, so crucial to pick nutrient-dense, healthy meals to help your breast milk production. Plus, eating nutritious meals after may help you feel better both psychologically and physically – and who doesn't want that?

Get to know the breast milk essentials

You may be asking why it's so crucial that you maintain a healthy, nutrient-dense diet when nursing.

In addition to improving your general health, a nutritious diet is vital for ensuring that your kid is receiving all the nutrients they need to flourish.

Except for vitamin D, breast milk provides everything your baby needs for optimal growth throughout the first 6 months.

But if your general diet does not supply adequate nutrients, it may damage both the quality of your breast milk and your health.

Research suggests that breast milk is made up of 87 percent water, 3.8 percent fat, 1.0 percent protein, and 7 percent carbohydrate and supplies 60 to 75 kcal/100ml.

Unlike infant formula, the calorie quantity and composition of breast milk vary. Breast milk fluctuates with each feeding and during your lactation phase, to satisfy the demands of your infant.

At the beginning of a feeding, the milk is more watery and generally quenches the baby's thirst. The milk that arrives later (hindmilk) is thicker, richer in fat, and more nutritious.

In reality, according to an earlier 2005 research, this milk may include 2 to 3 times as much fat as milk at the beginning of a feeding and 7 to 11 more calories per ounce. Therefore, to get the most nutritious milk, your infant must empty one breast before moving to the other.

Shoot for nutrient-dense nursing foods

There's a reason why your hunger levels may be at an all-time high while nursing your new baby. Creating breast milk is taxing on the body and needs additional total calories, as well as increased quantities of certain nutrients.

It's believed that your energy demands while nursing rise by roughly 500 calories per day. The demand for certain nutrients, including protein, vitamin D, vitamin A, vitamin E, vitamin C, B12, selenium, and zinc go rises as well.

This is why eating a range of nutrient-dense, whole foods are so vital for your health and your baby's health. Choosing meals rich in the aforementioned nutrients may help guarantee that you obtain all the macro- and micronutrients you and your little one need.

Here are some healthful and enjoyable meal options to emphasize while breastfeeding:

- Fish and seafood: salmon, seaweed, shellfish, sardines
- Meat and poultry: chicken, beef, lamb, hog, organ meats (such as liver) (such as liver)
- Fruits and vegetables: berries, tomatoes, bell peppers, cabbage, kale, garlic, broccoli
- Nuts and seeds: almonds, walnuts, chia seeds, hemp seeds, flaxseeds
- Healthy fats: avocados, olive oil, coconut, eggs, full-fat yogurt
- Fiber-rich starches: potatoes, butternut squash, sweet potatoes, beans, lentils, oats, quinoa, buckwheat
- Other foods: tofu, dark chocolate, kimchi, sauerkraut

We're love this list so far, but nursing moms are not restricted to these items.

And although having your favorite meals on occasion is healthy, it's ideal to decrease your consumption of processed foods like fast food and sugary morning cereals as much as possible. Instead, pick more healthful ones.

For example, if you're accustomed to beginning your day with a huge bowl of brightly colored breakfast cereal, consider substituting it with a bowl of oats topped with berries, unsweetened coconut, and a dab of nut butter for a satisfying and nutritious food source.

Adjust your nursing diet for both nutritional groups

Okay, so now that you have the fundamentals down of why eating nutrient-dense foods is vital while nursing, let's delve a little further into why it's necessary to pay particular attention to certain vitamins and minerals, too.

The nutrients in breast milk may be divided into two classes, based on the amount to which they are released into your milk.

If you're deficient in any group 1 nutrients, they won't secrete into your breast milk as quickly. So, supplementing with these nutrients may offer a tiny boost to their concentration in breast milk and promote the health of your kid as a consequence. (Got questions about vitamin supplements during pregnancy? Check-in with your doctor and check also the part below.)

On the other side, the quantity of group 2 nutrients in breast milk does not rely on how much mom takes in, thus supplementing won't improve your breast milk's nutritional content. Even so, these may still promote maternal health by restoring nutritional storage.

If all of that seems a bit complicated, no worries. Here's the bottom line: obtaining enough group 1 nutrient is crucial for both you and your baby, whereas getting enough group 2 nutrients is primarily simply necessary for you.

Group 1 nutrients

Here are the group 1 nutrients and how to find them in some typical dietary sources:

- Vitamin B1 (Thiamin): fish, pork, seeds, nuts, beans
- Vitamin B2 (Riboflavin): cheese, almonds, nuts, red meat, oily fish, eggs
- Vitamin B6: chickpeas, nuts, fish, poultry, potatoes, bananas, dried fruit
- Vitamin B12: shellfish, liver, yogurt, oily fish, nutritional yeast, eggs, crab, shrimp
- Choline: eggs, beef liver, chicken liver, fish, peanuts

- Vitamin A: sweet potatoes, carrots, dark leafy greens, organ meats, eggs
- Vitamin D: cod liver oil, oily fish, some mushrooms, fortified foods
- Selenium: Brazil nuts, seafood, turkey, whole wheat, seeds
- Iodine: dried seaweed, cod, milk, iodized salt

Group 2 nutrients

Here are the group 2 nutrients and some typical dietary sources:

- Folate: beans, lentils, leafy greens, asparagus, avocados
- Calcium: milk, yogurt, cheese, leafy greens, legumes

- Iron: red meat, pork, poultry, seafood, beans, green vegetables, dried fruit
- Copper: shellfish, whole grains, nuts, beans, organ meats, potatoes
- Zinc: oysters, red meat, poultry, beans, nuts, dairy

As we touched on before, the concentration of group 2 nutrients in breast milk are generally unaffected by your food consumption or body stockpiles.

So, if your intake is low, your body will remove these nutrients from your bone and tissue reserves to release them into your breast milk.

Your kid will always receive the proper quantity (hooray!), but your bodily reserves will get depleted if you don't obtain enough levels from your food. To prevent being deficient, these nutrients must come from your food or supplementation.

Consider taking supplements

Although a good diet is the most crucial element when it comes to nutrition during nursing, no doubt taking some supplements may assist restore your stocks of key vitamins and minerals.

There are a variety of reasons why new parents may be deficient in specific nutrients, including not eating the correct meals and the increased energy needs of breast milk production, combined with caring for your infant.

Taking supplements may help enhance your intake of key nutrients. But it's vital to be wary when picking supplements, as many include herbs and other ingredients that aren't healthy for nursing parents.

We've put together a list of vital nutrients for nursing women and aiding postpartum recovery in general. Always be careful to buy items from renowned companies that undergo testing by third-party agencies, like NSF or USP.

Multivitamins

A multivitamin may be a wonderful alternative for improving your consumption of key vitamins and minerals.

It's typical for women to be deficient in vitamins and minerals after birth and research reveal that deficits don't discriminate, impacting mothers in both high- and low-income situations.

For this reason, it may be a good idea to take a daily multivitamin, particularly if you don't believe you're receiving enough vitamins and minerals via your food alone. (With so much to worry about as a new parent, who is?)

Vitamin B-12

Vitamin B-12 is an extremely vital water-soluble vitamin that is crucial for your baby's health, as well as your health, while nursing.

Plus, many women — notably those following largely plant-based diets, those who've had gastric bypass surgery, and those who are on specific medicines (such as acid reflux meds) — are already at an elevated risk of having low B-12 levels.

If you belong to one of these groups, or if you believe that you don't consume enough B-12-rich foods like fish, meat, poultry, eggs, and fortified foods, then taking a B-complex or B-12 supplement is a smart option.

Keep in mind that most high-quality multivitamins and prenatal supplements have enough B-12 to meet your requirements.

Omega-3 (DHA)

Omega-3 fats are all the rage today and for good reason. These lipids, naturally abundant in fatty fish and algae, serve critical functions in both maternal and fetal health.

For example, the omega-3 lipid DHA is crucial for the development of your baby's nervous system, skin, and eyes. Plus, the content of this essential fat in breast milk significantly relies on your dietary levels.

What's more, research reveals that newborns who are given breast milk with high amounts of DHA have superior eyesight and neurodevelopment results.

Because breast milk concentrations of omega-3s mirror your diet of these critical fats, it's crucial that you receive enough. We suggest that nursing moms take 250 to 375 mg daily of DHA with EPA, another vital omega-3 lipid.

Although eating 8 to 12 ounces of fish, particularly fatty fish like salmon and sardines, will help you meet the recommended dietary levels, taking a fish oil or krill oil supplement is a practical approach to satisfy your daily requirements.

Vitamin D

Vitamin D is exclusively present in a few foods, notably fatty fish, fish liver oils, and fortified goods. Your body may also make it through sunlight exposure, albeit it depends on numerous things, such as skin color and where you reside.

Research suggests that it performs several critical functions in your body and is crucial for immune function and bone health.

Vitamin D is normally only available in low concentrations in breast milk, particularly when sun exposure is restricted.

Therefore, supplementing with 400 IU of vitamin D per day is suggested for breastfed newborns and babies eating less than 1 liter of formula per day, beginning within the first few days of life and continuing until they are 12 months of age, according to the American Academy of Pediatrics.

According to a study, supplementing with 6,400 IU daily may help provide your kid with enough quantities of vitamin D via breast milk alone. Interestingly, this quantity is substantially greater than the current recommended vitamin D consumption of 600 IU for nursing parents.

Vitamin D insufficiency is highly frequent amongst nursing moms. And insufficiency may lead to unfavorable health effects, including an increased risk of postpartum depression. That's why supplementing with this vitamin is suggested.

Ask your healthcare professional for exact dose recommendations depending on your current vitamin D levels.

Drink lots of water

In addition to being hungrier than normal when nursing, you may feel thirstier as well.

When your infant latches onto your breast, your oxytocin levels surge. This stimulates your milk to start flowing. This also promotes thirst and helps ensure that you keep well hydrated when feeding your baby.

It's crucial to understand that your water requirements may vary based on things like exercise levels and nutritional consumption. There's no one-size-fits-all rule when it comes to how much liquids you need while nursing.

As a matter of thumb, you should always drink when you are thirsty and until you have satisfied your thirst.

But if you feel particularly exhausted, dizzy, or as if your milk supply is dropping, you may need to drink extra water. The greatest method to know whether you are drinking enough water is the color and smell of your urine.

If it is dark yellow and has a strong stench, it's an indication that you're dehydrated and need to drink more water.

Foods and beverages to avoid when breastfeeding

Although you may have heard differently, it's acceptable to consume just about any meal while nursing, unless you have an allergy to a particular item.

And, while certain tastes from food, spices, or drinks may modify the taste of your breast milk, research suggests it's unlikely that this would influence your baby's feeding time or make them cranky.

Another popular misunderstanding is that "gassy" vegetables like cauliflower and cabbage may promote gassiness in your infant, too. Although these meals may make you gassy, the gas-promoting components do not pass to breast milk, citing a 2017 study.

In summary, most foods and beverages are healthy while nursing, but there is a handful that should be restricted or avoided. If you suspect anything may be harming your infant badly, contact your healthcare professional for guidance.

Caffeine

About 1 percent of the caffeine you ingest is passed to breast milk, and studies suggest it takes newborns far longer to break down caffeine. Drinking caffeinated drinks like coffee has not been found to cause damage, although they may disrupt the baby's sleep.

Therefore, it's suggested that nursing mothers restrict their coffee consumption to around 2 to 3 cups per day. It's a disappointment, we know, but at least some coffee is permitted, right?

Alcohol

Alcohol may also find its way into breast milk. The concentration mirrors the quantity present in the mother's blood. However, newborns metabolize alcohol at only half the rate of adults.

Nursing after consuming only 1 to 2 drinks might lower your baby's milk intake by up to 23 percent and cause irritability and poor sleep.

Because alcohol use too close to nursing might significantly affect your baby's healthy, the AAP recommends alcohol intake should be minimized while breastfeeding.

The AAP recommended no more than 0.5 grams of alcohol per kilogram of body weight, which for a 60-kilogram (132-pound) mother, equals 2 ounces of liquor, 8 ounces of wine, or 2 beers.

Although it's totally fine to have an alcoholic beverage as a nursing parent, it's advisable to wait at least 2 hours after drinking to breastfeed your infant.

Cow's milk

Although unusual. Some newborns may be allergic to cow's milk. And if your infant has a cow's milk allergy, you must remove all dairy items from your diet.

Up to 1 percent of breastfed newborns are allergic to cow's milk protein from their mother's diet and may have rashes, dermatitis, diarrhea, bloody stools, vomiting, or baby colic.

Your healthcare professional may provide you guidance on how long to avoid dairy from your diet, and when it's okay to reintroduce dairy.

Breastfeeding and weight loss

You may be tempted to lose weight rapidly after delivery, but weight reduction takes time and it's crucial to be nice to your body throughout this transition.

With the multiple hormonal changes that take place during nursing and the calorie requirement of creating breast milk, you may have a larger appetite during breastfeeding.

Restricting calories too much, particularly during the first several months of nursing, may lower your milk production and much-needed energy levels.

Fortunately, nursing alone has been demonstrated to promote weight reduction, particularly when sustained for 6 months or longer. (That said, losing weight when nursing doesn't happen for everyone!)

Losing roughly 1.1 pounds (0.5 kilograms) each week with a mix of a balanced diet and exercise should not alter your milk production or milk composition, providing that you are not undernourished, to begin with.

All nursing women, irrespective of their weight, should take appropriate calories.

But if you're underweight, you'll probably be more sensitive to calorie restriction.

For this reason, women with less body weight must eat more calories to prevent a decline in milk production.

All in all, remember that reducing weight after delivery is a marathon, not a sprint. It took months to put on the weight for a healthy pregnancy for both you and your kid, and it may take you months to drop it — and that's alright.

The most essential thing to remember while attempting to reduce pregnancy weight is that restrictive diets are not healthy for general health and don't effective for long-term weight reduction.

Following a balanced diet, including exercise in your daily routine, and getting adequate sleep are the greatest strategies to encourage healthy weight reduction.

In Summary

Breastfeeding is a hard effort! Your body demands extra calories and nutrients to keep you and your baby fed and healthy.

If you're not consuming enough calories or nutrient-rich meals, this might significantly influence the quality of your breast milk. It might also be damaging to your health.

It's more vital than ever to consume a range of healthful, nutritious meals and minimize processed junk. Avoid excess coffee and alcohol usage, and stick to the recommended intakes to keep your kid healthy.

If you need to, make sure to integrate supplements into your regimens, such as vitamin D and omega-3s. And lastly, be patient with your body. Take it one day at a time and remind yourself every day how amazing you are.

www.ingramcontent.com/pod-product-compliance
Lightning Source LLC
Chambersburg PA
CBHW051556250726
48653CB00004BA/1187